# POWER MAX
# TRANSFORMATION

# Method

# POWER MAX TRANSFORMATION

# Method

**The Best Isotonic Exercises to build muscle, increase strength, burn fat and sculpt the best body without the use of weights!**

**BECOME POWERFUL!**

The Power Max Transformation Method was written to help you get closer to your physical potential when it comes to real muscle sculpting strengthening exercises. The exercises and routines in this book are quite demanding, so consult your physician and have a physical exam taken prior to the start of this exercise program. Proceed with the suggested exercises and information at your own risk. The Publishers and author shall not be liable or responsible for any loss, injury, or damage allegedly arising from the information or suggestions in this book.

Power Max Transformation Method
muscle-building Course

By

Birch Tree Publishing
Published by Birch Tree Publishing

Power Max Transformation Method
Published in 2019, All rights reserved,
No part of this book may be reproduced, scanned,
or distributed in any printed or electronic form without permission.

Birch Tree Publishing

# Dedication

For my lovely wife Mel and business partner, this book is for **YOU!**

# Contents

**Introduction:** STEVE FARR'S MUSCLE TRANSFORMATION    **PG 7**

**Chapter 1:** MUSCLE FIBER ANALYSIS    **PG 12**

**Chapter 2:** SCULPT A POWERFUL CHEST    **PG 15**

**Chapter 3: DEVELOP BARN DOOR SHOULDERS**    **PG 18**

**Chapter 4: DEVELOP A POWERFUL V-TAPER**    **PG 23**

**Chapter 5: DEVELOP POWERFUL NECK MUSCLES**    **PG 31**

**Chapter 6: BUILD BASEBALL SHAPED BICEPS**    **PG 35**

**Chapter 7: DEVELOP DYNAMITE TRICEPS**    **PG 41**

**Chapter 8: DEVELOP RIPPED FOREARMS**    **PG 47**

**Chapter 9: LEGS/LOWER BACK HAMSTRINGS**    **PG 50**

**Chapter 10: CALVES**    **PG 62**

**Chapter 11: DEVELOP RIPPED ABS**    **PG 65**

**Chapter 12:** ULTIMATE 20,10,5 DENSITY PROGRAM    **PG 71**

**Chapter 13:** ULTIMATE MUSCLE BUILDING ACCELERATION PROGRAM    **PG 83**

**Chapter 14:** ENHANCING MUSCLE FIBER ACTIVATION    **PG 87**

**Chapter 15:** THE ISOMETRIC POWER MAX PROGRAM    **PG 103**

**Chapter 16:** THE ISOMETRIC 10,10,10 PROGRAM    **PG 125**

**Chapter 17: Isometric Power Contraction Program**    **PG 134**

# Today Finally "GET" RIPPED

## And now, the worlds fastest muscle-building program is in the palms of your hands!

## Introduction by Marlon Birch and Steve Farr

Steve Farr has been in touch with me since mid 2006 and soon after became one of my beta-test subject for my various muscle-building programs, a self resistance weight gaining master-plan. It was the first time he was introduced to self resistance an exercise program where you resist with the other limb. For example, performing a curl with the right arm, while the left adds resistance while you perform a full range motion.

Steve gained a serious 10 plus pounds in a short period of time, a lot of his gains happened within week 7 of the third muscle building phase.  He trained using a full-body plan for the first 3 weeks. Working his neck, shoulders, arms and calves on the other days. On week seven, Steve changed his bodypart hits to, every-other-day, using a split routine, alternating the bodyparts. Steve's quest to gain strength, muscle and power is quite interesting, and inspiring, so I will let Steve fill you in on that one.....

Growing up like most teenagers I started lifting weights and doing martial arts. Plus I wanted to become the most powerful and muscular guy on the planet as well. I also had dreams of some day looking like a bodybuilder and follow the sport of bodybuilding. However, after lifting weights for a few years I gained a lot of strength but, no real size gains came. I later was told about steriods and how it is the "magic" cure to massive muscles and might.

I refused to resort to those lengths and continued lifting weights anyway. While I did make improvements with my physique, I did not look like a guy that was working out regardless of what I did. So I decided perhaps this is not for me. . the real size I was seeking didn't materialize. So I stopped lifting weights altogether, life moved on and gradually I became a very soft 220 pounder, with some bad habits.

In 2006  I decided to search the internet and find a way to get back in shape. "As chance would have it, I made contact with a guy I saw online on one of the forums. His name was Marlon Birch. He told me that he's been a lifelong Charles Atlas student and he used dynamic tension exercises to build his body. Plus he developed various training systems that increase muscle size without lifting weights or using machines. I thought to myself, GREAT I'm in!

Finally, I thought..... I can develop the body of my dreams with the help of this guy. Plus Marlon wanted me to do things a certain way to achieve that goal so, this motivated me even more to stay the course. So I tried my best and followed all the exercises as he layed them out. I never missed a single workout, I was focused, motivated and excited to see what I would look like after it all. Within this book you will see the programs that I used.

The progress, not to mention the muscles really started to pile on with the routines. I could not believe my eyes. After all those years of spinning my heels with weights, there was a much faster, and better way for me to add layers of muscle within a few short months. I am now successfully building more and more muscle each month by refining my bodypart exercises within a phase approach. As well as various stress and hy-brid methods that I have learned from Marlon.

Now today, I can safely say, I am achieving the physique I have always dreamed of having. Today I am doing a hy-brid program from Marlon that will decrease my bodyfat levels and gain more muscle to a hard as nails, ripped 200 pounds. His new innovations, has already got me to the point I am sold by the guy. However, I am striving to become far better than I am now. This book is about transforming your body, mind and spirit, which is what health, strength and physique enhancement is all about.
I am really excited and positive to say that once you try the programs in the book, you will make some of the best gains you've ever made. Maybe far greater than I ever have.

Join the men and women that are already using my body transformation books and pro-grams with great success. **GET TRANSFORMED** today.

Keep moving forward

*Yours In Health and Strength*
*Marlon Birch and Steve Farr*

# LET'S BEGIN

# LET'S BEGIN

If you are reading this book, you already appreciate the importance of exercising for health, strength and well being. The Power Max Transformation Method will turn you into a powerful well built man. Let's face it, being a great success at exercising means constant practice to transform yourself to become the best you can be.

Of course, when it comes to training-like most everything else in life-sometimes circumstances seem to get in the way from allowing you to exercise. Now, thanks to The Power Max Method, you will always get a great workout-no matter where you are.

Resistance strength training with the Power Max Method enhances:

1) Resistance strength training stimulates muscles to burn more calories than anything else. After your workout your metabolism is triggered for 40 hours after the session.
2) Your body will take on a different shape, and your clothes will fit far better.
3) Your flexibility will increase and resistance training will keep you young.
4) Your bones will become stronger. We lose bone mass as we get older, but resistance strength training increases bone density and add greater strength.
5) A stronger and healthy heart with enhanced blood flow.
6) Stress levels will be reduced due to exercise.
7) Resistance strength training also creates better sleeping patterns.
8) "No need to get depressed". Regular resistance training will ward off symptoms of depression.
9) Mental sharpness will be developed. This takes place due resistance training decreasing blood levels of homocysteine, the protein that's linked to developing Alzheimer's and dementia. Plus, resistance training enhances cognitive function. Workouts will improve memory and you will have longer attention spans.
10) Develop lazar-like focus.

# The Training Program that will create

## a

# Powerful

# Ripped Body

# Chapter 1:
# MUSCLE FIBER ANALYSIS

How strength training increase strength, help you lose bodyfat and develop a great build.

## Create the body of your dreams anytime

# 01 MUSCLE FIBER ANALYSIS

With my training under Marlon Birch, I've realised there are so many so-called theories floating around, it's hard to separate muscle-building fact from fiction. For many years, it was gospel that fast twitch 2Bs were best for muscle growth.

These were the supposedly **GET BIG** fibers. The true **KINGS** to muscle growth are the type 2As—the fibers that are fast-twitch, with an endurance element. This however, gives the trainee a double **BOOM** with a size and conditioning effect. Once done correctly.

Plus guess work does not exist within these pages. Marlon has taken all of that out by his muscle-building experience with loads of trial and error. Our rep range and methods stimulate and develop the important endurance fast twitch fibers that is important for enhancing muscle growth and strength gains.

Our program stress the muscles being worked to it's maximum and not the tendons. Critical development from endurance-oriented fibers do not occur unless you keep tension time, and the length of the set, at 30 seconds and beyond.

2A fibers have both endurance and anaerobic capabilities, so to get the most growth you need to tax both facets of the muscle for optimum size gains. So will a low rep range build any muscle at all? Low reps do build muscle, but growth is slow and limited until the endurance-oriented capacities are taxed. This then stimulates the 2A fast-twitch fibers which promote muscle growth.

This is why the trainee need to stay within the 15-20 rep range mark, this increases the load time placed on the fibers for serious growth and development to occur. 30 plus seconds will coax the size principal where low-threshold units are called first to fire, followed by the mediums, then the high threshold units. This is the best way to stimulate many fiber types to fire rapidly. However, most importantly, the aerobic component of the fast twitch fibers will be called into place promoting more muscle growth.

# 01 MUSCLE FIBER ANALYSIS

Our programs are designed to activate endurance fast twitch 2As, and extend the capacity in the ones that are firing rapidly. This however makes the set 10 times more effective at promoting optimum muscle increase. Priming the nervous system and stimulating more blood blockage which expands the internal structures of the muscle cell. So in short, low reps do not tax the fast twitch fibers enough to stimulate optimum muscle growth.

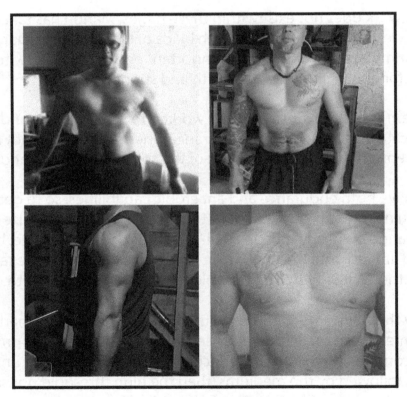

A few shots of Steve and his progress

# Chapter 2:

# CHEST

## SCULPT A POWERFUL CHEST

# SCULPT A POWERFUL CHEST

## 02  SCULPT A POWERFUL CHEST

The chest muscles allow you to push or move the arm forward or across the body. These muscles are activated in any throwing or pushing motion. Aesthetically, building a powerful chest is a sign of power in men.

However the chest muscles are not used on a daily basis, so most times they are under developed. So despite,the simplicity of how these muscles contract, they can be trained in a number of various angles of push and pull, each offer its own special muscle enhancing properties.

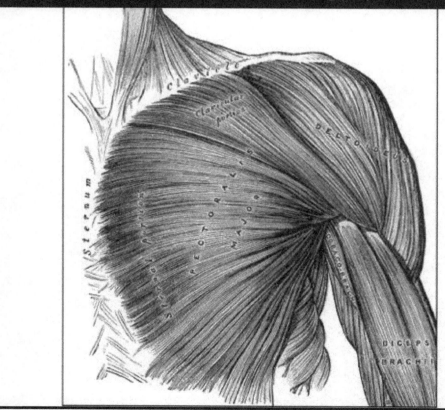

## CHEST EXERCISES

# 02 SCULPT A POWERFUL CHEST

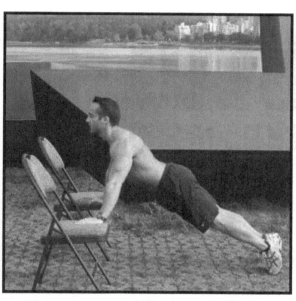

### INCLINE PUSHUPS

This exercise is the Granddaddy of all upper-body exercises. It's the best upper-body builder and conditioner there is. This exercise is performed exactly as shown.

Place your hands on two chairs that are 15 inches high, the higher you go the greater pre-stretch there is. At the bottom position to enhance muscle-building stimuli pause at the bottom for 2-3 seconds before reversing the movement.

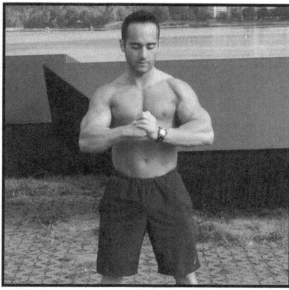

### LIEDERMAN PRESS

This is an awesome building and shaping movement. Works the entire chest as well as the shoulders and triceps musculature. Start off with the hands in the middle or the armpit.

Press right palm against the left palm towards the left armpit.

Pause for 1-2 seconds and press the arm back to the other armpit, pause again before repeating.

# Chapter 3:

# SHOULDERS
## DEVELOP BARN DOOR SHOULDERS

# DEVELOP BARN DOOR SHOULDERS

## 03 DEVELOP BARN DOOR SHOULDERS

The shoulder muscles are divided into three heads and are quite unique and move the arm in all directions. The front muscle raises the arm for ward, the side muscles made up of variable number of muscle bundles, and raises the arm out to the sides. The rear or posterior muscle, is designed to pull the arm backwards. Upright rows is a multi-muscle-use exercise, which is a compound exercise. This exercise recruits the front and side heads of the shoulders that tie in well with stimulating the upper and mid-back muscles as well giving the entire girdle complete development.

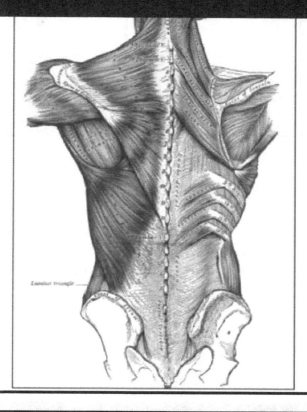

## SHOULDER EXERCISES

## 03 DEVELOP BARN DOOR SHOULDERS

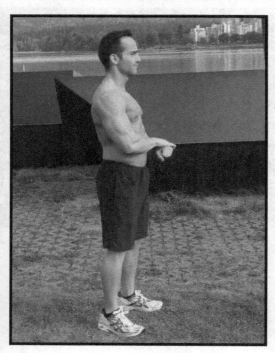 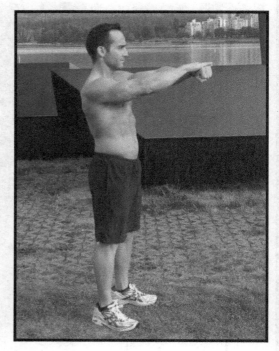

### FORWARD RAISES

Grasp the right hand with the left in front of the body as shown. Gradually raise the arm forward against the resistance of the other hand. Switch arms and continue. This works the front shoulder muscles.

## SHOULDER EXERCISES

# 03 DEVELOP BARN DOOR SHOULDERS

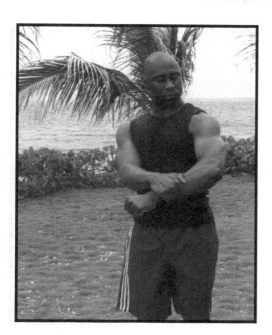 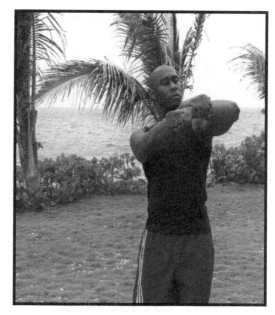

## LATERAL RAISES

Grasp the left arm that is across the body as in the picture. Now raise the arm outwards towards the side contracted position resisting with the right arm.

## SHOULDER EXERCISES

## 03 DEVELOP BARN DOOR SHOULDERS

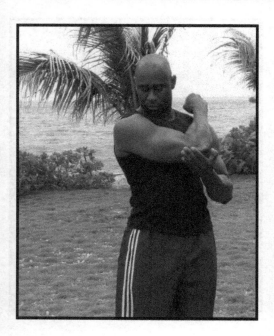 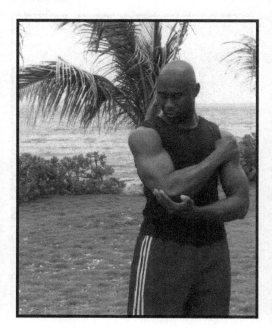

### ACROSS THE BODY PULLS

Bring the right elbow across the chest and grasp the left elbow with a firm grip. Slowly force the right elbow across the body towards the right hip resisting with the left hand. This exercise adds strength and development to the rear shoulder muscles and upper back.

# Chapter 4:

# UPPER BACK

## DEVELOP A POWERFUL V-TAPER

# DEVELOP A POWERFUL V-TAPER

## 04 DEVELOP A POWERFUL V-TAPER

The entire back is made up of numerous muscles overlapping each other. Most trainees find the back quite difficult to fully develop. The reason? As the saying goes, out of sight, out of mind. We cannot directly see the back muscles, plus we cannot see it flex like we would see the biceps.

We make training the entire back musculature much easier making developing the back obviously simple once you know what you are doing, you can bring these muscles up to speed. We are looking at the large Latissimus that covers the majority of the back. The trapezius is broken up into two sections.

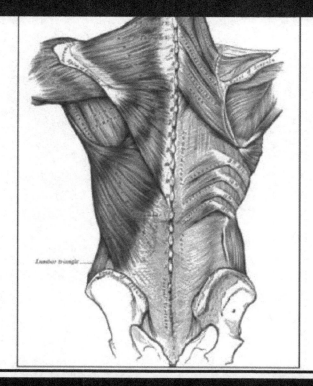

## UPPER BACK EXERCISES

# 04  DEVELOP A POWERFUL V-TAPER

## DO NOT NEGLECT THE MID AND LOWER TRAPS

The upper traps and mid-back muscles. Plus we have the teres major, which is strongly stimulated with unilateral work, which makes self resistance the ideal movement. The infraspinatus muscle is like a half circle on each side of the upper back and is a very important rotator cuff muscle.

This muscle stabilize the shoulder and prevent dislocations. Even though this muscle is at the back, most traditional exercises do not fully target these muscles. However with self resistance there are exercises that target this area for full development.

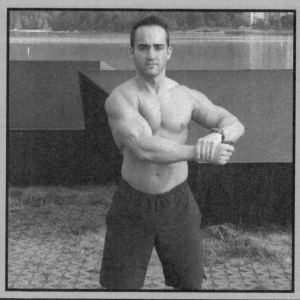

## UPPER BACK EXERCISES

## 04 DEVELOP A POWERFUL V-TAPER

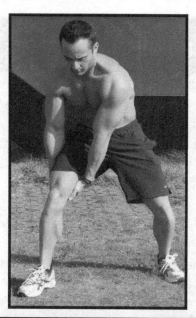 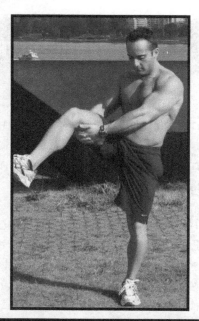

## ANOTHER VERSION TO HIT THIGH ROWS

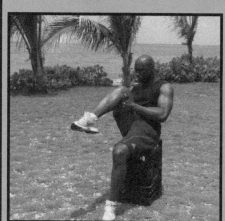

Interlock the fingers behind the knee as shown with right leg. With both arms pull the thigh upwards towards the chest while resisting with the leg. If balance is an issue perform the exercise seated.

## UPPER BACK EXERCISES

## 04 DEVELOP A POWERFUL V-TAPER

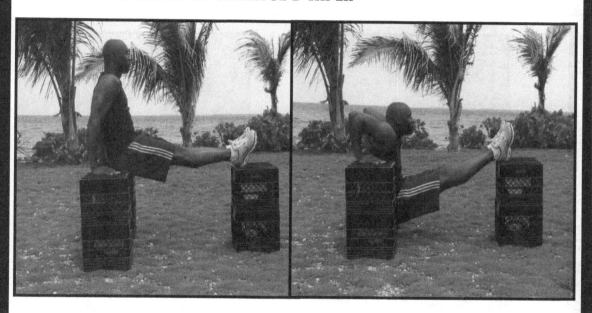

## THREE CHAIR DIPS

As shown place each hand at least 15-16 inches apart, or shoulder width. Lower the body between the chairs pause one second and reverse the movement to the starting position. **Maintain a slight bend in the elbow at the top position.** This is an awesome upper back widener.

## UPPER BACK EXERCISES

## 04 DEVELOP A POWERFUL V-TAPER

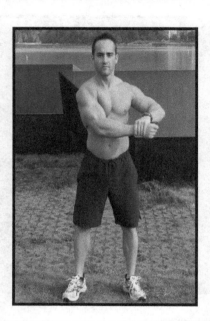 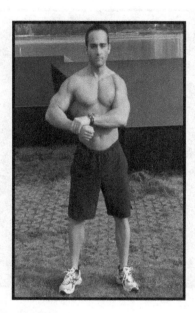

### ACROSS THE BODY ROWS

Bring your right arm across the body pre-stretching the mid-back, grasp the wrist with the left hand. Slowly pull the arm across the body toward the right armpit against the resistance supplied by the left hand. Repeat the move ment then switch arms. This adds thickens to the mid back and lats, along with the rear part of the shoulders.

## UPPER BACK EXERCISES

## 04 DEVELOP A POWERFUL V-TAPER

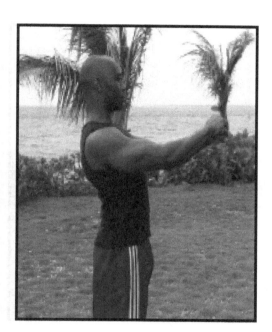 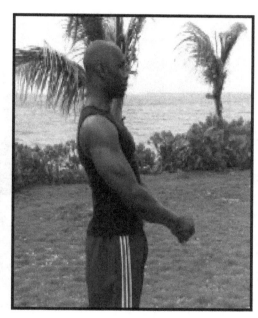

### STIFF ARM PULLDOWNS

Grasp the left hand with the right as in the picture. Gradually pull the arm downwards while resisting with the bottom arm. At finished position repeat by pressing the bottom arm up again by resisting against the top hand. Resisting in both directions for reps, then switch. Fantastic Upper and mid-back strengthener.

## UPPER BACK EXERCISES

## 04 DEVELOP A POWERFUL V-TAPER

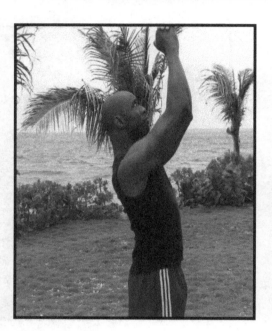 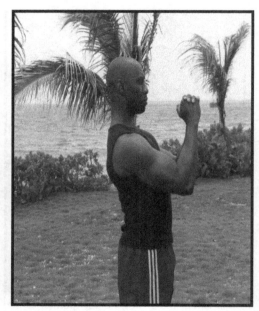

## ANOTHER VERSION TO HIT THE POWERFUL UPPER BACK

With the arms over-head place your left hand on top of the right fist as shown. Pull down with the left hand resisting with the right, once at finished position press the right hand up resisting with the left hand for the desired reps. Then switch arms.

# Chapter 5:

# TRAPS/NECK

## DEVELOP POWERFUL NECK MUSCLES

# DEVELOP POWERFUL TRAPS

## 05 DEVELOP POWERFUL TRAPS/MID-BACK

The trapezuis muscles are in three parts: The upper traps, this lifts the shoulder girdle, the (bottom-traps, which works in opposition to the upper traps. Lowers the shoulders. The middle traps (mid-back) which along with the rhomboids that partially covers, bring the shoulder blades together.
With the self resistance and isometrics the upper traps will look impressive in clothes and will add a complete look to your upper body. Making it more balanced. The self resistance method of exercise will avoid imbalances between the upper and mid-trap muscles. Complete develop-ment takes place due to an efficient training program.

A lot of our various exercises stimulate various sections of the muscles. Which prevents an imbalance of the upper traps becoming far too developed than the mid-back and lower-traps muscles. It's important to know that the lower traps stabilize and protect the shoulder girdle.

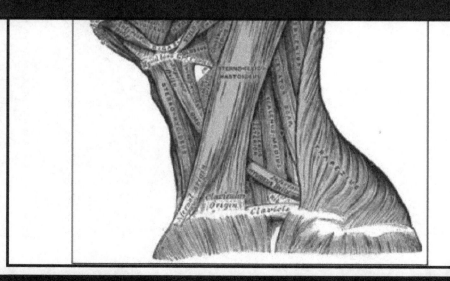

## TRAPEZUIS EXERCISES

## 05 DEVELOP POWERFUL TRAPS/MID-BACK

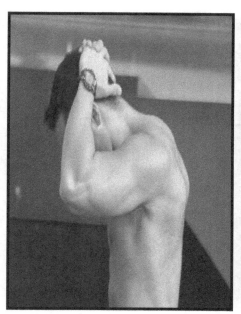 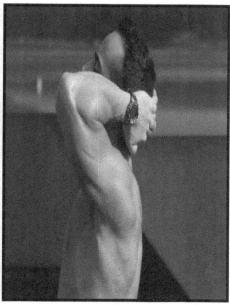

## REAR NECK PRESS

Place your hands behind your head and tuck the chin on the upper chest as shown. Now press the head against the hand while resisting with the hand until you're looking straight up. Use a light tension at the beginning and increase the tension to medium as you get stronger and more conditioned.

## TRAPEZUIS EXERCISES

## 05 DEVELOP POWERFUL TRAPS/MID-BACK

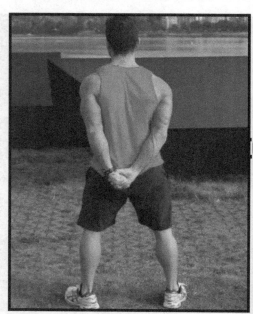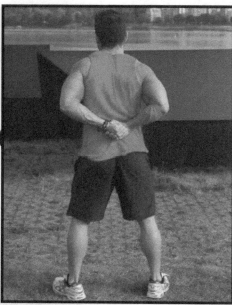

## REVERSE UPRIGHT ROW

Place your arm behind your back as shown. Hold onto the wrist with the other hand lean forward a-little and pull the right arm upwards while resisting with the right hand.

This works the mid-back, upper traps and rear delts.

# Chapter 6:

# BICEPS

## BUILD BASEBALL SHAPED BICEPS

# BUILD BASEBALL SHAPED BICEPS

## 06 BUILD BASEBALL SHAPED BICEPS

The biceps muscle has two heads. A short head, which is on the inside of the arm, and a long head, which is on the outside. This is the part that people see first. The main roll of the biceps is to flex the forearm, by bringing the hand towards the shoulder. In order to build powerful complete biceps, you need to learn that the biceps do not work by itself.

The brachialis, which is under the bicep when developed gives the bicep a larger and fuller appearance. Performing curls place undesirable tension on the tendon near the elbow. In other words, the biceps are placed in a very vulnerable position. Always start all bicep exercises with a slight bend at the start and finish. Always maintain tension on the biceps and not the joint.

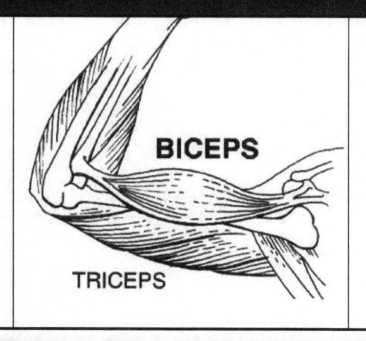

BICEPS

TRICEPS

## BICEP EXERCISES

## 06 BUILD BASEBALL SHAPED BICEPS

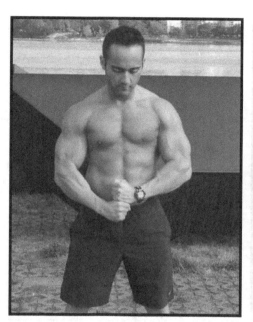
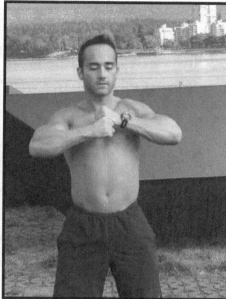

## HAMMER CURLS

A great Bicep/Forearm combo. Place the wrists as shown in the picture above. Now pull with the right hand or bottom hand upwards to the chest while resisting with the top hand.

At upper chest level reverse the exercise by pressing the top wrist down and resisting with the bottom wrist. Repeat for reps then switch arms.

## BICEP EXERCISES

## 06 BUILD BASEBALL SHAPED BICEPS

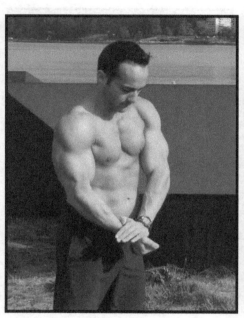 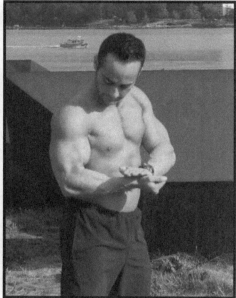

## PALM UP CURLS

Grasp your right wrist with the left hand. Pull the right arm up ward towards the shoulder while resisting with the left hand. At the shoulder, reverse the exercise by pushing the left arm downwards resisting with the right.

## BICEP EXERCISES

## 06 BUILD BASEBALL SHAPED BICEPS

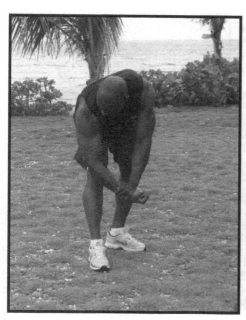
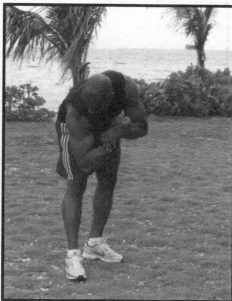

### CONCENTRATION CURLS

This is a great bicep finisher move. Peak contraction to hit that long head again. As pictured in start position hold on to the right wrist with left hand and pull the right arm towards the face while resisting with the left hand.

Now reverse the exercise by pushing the left arm down and resisting with the right. Complete your reps then switch arms and repeat movement.

## BICEP EXERCISES

# 06 BUILD BASEBALL SHAPED BICEPS

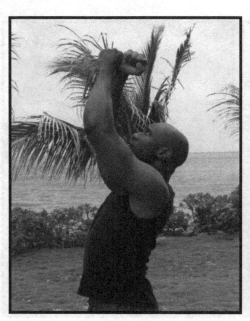 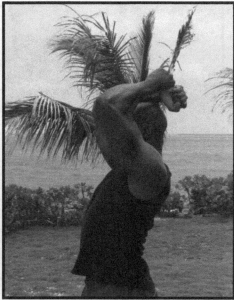

## OVER-HEAD CURLS

Make a fist with both hands place it above your head. Now pull the top fist downward while resisting with the bottom fist. At the bottom reverse the exercise by pushing upwards with the bottom fist while resisting with the top fist. Use a light to moderate tension due to the tricep tendons being quite sensitive at that position. **KEEP THE ELBOW BENT AT THE TOP**

# Chapter 7:

# TRICEPS
## DEVELOP DYNAMITE TRICEPS

# DEVELOP DYNAMITE TRICEPS

## 07 DEVELOP DYNAMITE TRICEPS

### DEVELOP DYNAMITE TRICEPS

The triceps has three heads: The lateral head, middle head and the long head. The role of the triceps is to straighten the arm. The triceps works in opposition to the biceps and brachialis muscles. The triceps has three heads this makes it much larger in mass than the biceps and the brachialis.

However unfortunately most pay attention to the biceps, leaving the triceps underdeveloped. The lateral head, which is on the outside is what people see first. The triceps are easy to develop and we have made it easy for the trainee to achieve this.

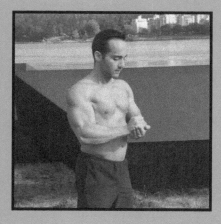

## TRICEP EXERCISES

# 07 DEVELOP DYNAMITE TRICEPS

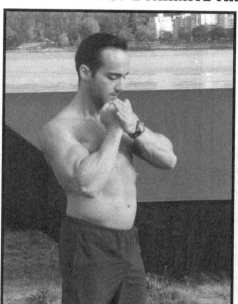 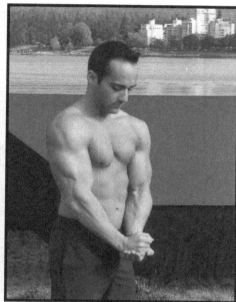

## SINGLE ARM PUSHDOWNS

As shown above, press the right arm downwards while resisting with the left hand. Resist on the downward stroke only.
**Do not straighten the elbow** At the contracted position at the bottom pause for 2 seconds then reverse the movement maintaining tension on the muscle. Perform your reps then switch arms.

## TRICEP EXERCISES

# 07 DEVELOP DYNAMITE TRICEPS

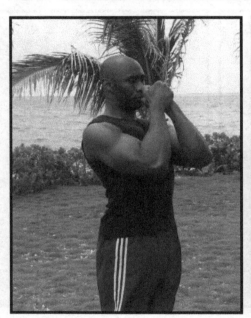
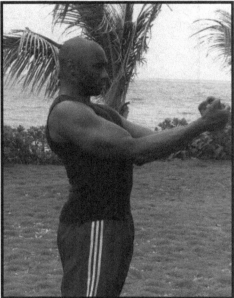

## FORWARD TRICEP EXTENSIONS

Place the left fist in the right hand. Now push the left hand for ward while resisting with the right hand. At the finished position reverse the movement by pulling the right hand towards you resisting with the left. **Do not straighten the elbow**

## TRICEP EXERCISES

# 07 DEVELOP DYNAMITE TRICEPS

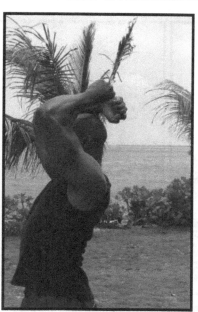 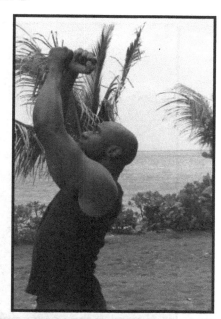

## OVERHEAD TRICEP EXTENSIONS

Make a fist with both hands place it behind your neck. Now press the bottom fist upward while resisting with the top fist. At the top reverse the exercise by pushing downwards with the top fist while resisting with the bottom fist. Use moderate tension due to the tricep tendons being quite sensitive at that position. **Do not straighten the elbow**

## TRICEP EXERCISES

# 07 DEVELOP DYNAMITE TRICEPS

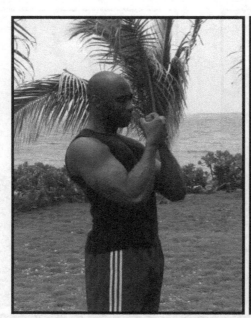 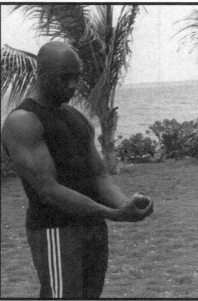

## REVERSE GRIP PRESSDOWN

Place the left fist palm up in the right hand. Now press the left hand downwards resisting with the right hand. Relax and repeat movement. **Do not straighten the elbow at the bottom position.**

# Chapter 8:

# FOREARMS
## DEVELOP RIPPED FOREARMS

# DEVELOP RIPPED FOREARMS

## 08 DEVELOP RIPPED FOREARMS

### DEVELOP RIPPED FOREARMS

#### DEVELOP POWERFUL FOREARMS

Forearm muscles are involved in every daily activity, just like the calves and abdominals. We use these muscles all the time, when we drive, write, type, hold a bag and even open a door.

Many of the muscles of the forearm deal with Muscle-multi-use. When you are moving the elbow by lowering and raising the forearm. Moving the wrist up and down by, raising and lowering the hand. All self resistance exercises stress the forearms to contract which will increase your grip strength.

## FOREARM EXERCISES

## 08 DEVELOP RIPPED FOREARMS

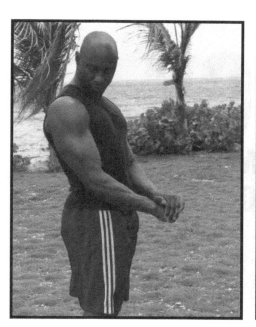 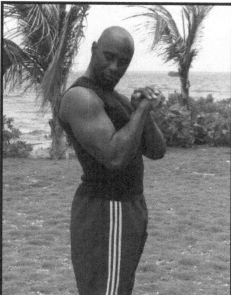

## REVERSE CURLS

This is the Grand-daddy of all exercises.A great bicep/forearm widener. Place the left hand on top of the right fist. Now pull the right hand upwards while resisting with the left hand.

Pause for 2 seconds, at the shoulder reverse the exercise by pushing the left arm down-wards resisting with the right hand. Repeat for reps then switch arms. This exercise adds fullness to the upper arms giving the bicep a fuller appearance.

# Chapter 9:

# LEGS
## DEVELOP POWERFUL TIRELESS LEGS/LOWERBACK

# DEVELOP POWERFUL TIRELESS LEGS

## 09 DEVELOP POWERFUL TIRELESS LEGS

### DEVELOP POWERFUL THIGHS

The thigh muscles are basically made up of four main muscles: the vastus lateral muscle, this is located on the outside of the thighs. The vastus medial muscle, this is located on the inside of the thigh muscles towards the knee.

Better known as the tear drop because of its shape. The recus-femoris, which is located in the center of the muscles, and the vastus intermedius, this muscle is mostly covered by all the other muscles of the thighs. The Power Isometric Isotonic Method will develop tireless thighs with a power pack punch.

## LEG EXERCISES

## 09 DEVELOP POWERFUL TIRELESS LEGS

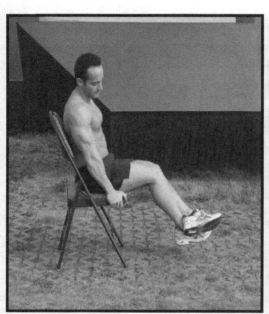 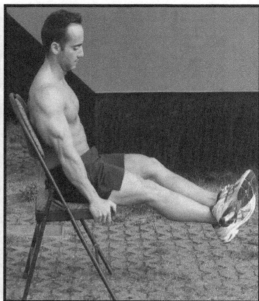

## LEG EXTENSIONS

While seated on a chair, box or stool, place the right leg over the left as shown in the picture. Now extend the left leg outwards resisting with the right. At the top pause for 2 seconds, then reverse the movement by pulling down the right while resisting with the left.
**DO NOT STRAIGHTEN THE KNEE**

## LEG EXERCISES

## 09 DEVELOP POWERFUL TIRELESS LEGS

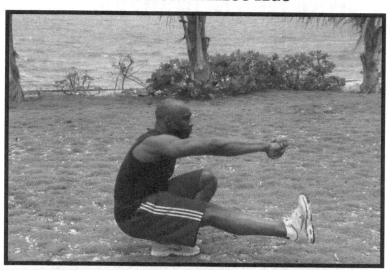

## ONE LEGGED SQUATS

A Few exercises are as impressive as a properly conducted one-leg-squat. Some of the best athletes and strength coaches in the world are unable to perform a single rep of this advanced exercise. Let alone a full set of them.

Stand with your knees slightly bent and your arms outstretched to balance. Lift one leg off the ground and place it as far-out in front of you as possible while keeping it straight. (don't worry you will get better in time). Then, slowly lower yourself as far as possible on your balancing leg.
When your hamstrings touch your calves (or as far as you can perform this exercise at first), push back up with the supporting leg to the start position and repeat. If your balance isn't tip top perform the exercise holding on to a chair with a free hand for support.

## LEG EXERCISES

## 09 DEVELOP POWERFUL TIRELESS LEGS

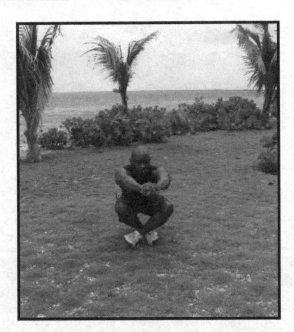

## CROSS FEET SQUATS

Another excellent exercise for the overall thigh and ham-strings. Start off as shown in the bottom position with feet crossed. Slowly under control push yourself to the finished position. **NO BOUNCING!**

One second pause then reverse the movement to the starting position. This exercise may be difficult at first but keep practicing and as night follows day it gets easier.

## LEG EXERCISES

## 09 DEVELOP POWERFUL TIRELESS LEGS

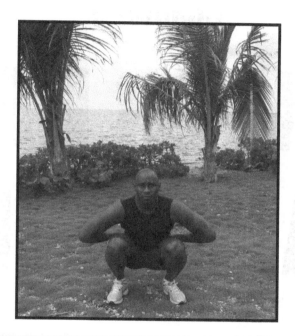

## REGULAR SQUATS

This is the easiest of body-weight exercises. Start off in the stand
ing position shows then lower yourself under control to the
finished position. Now reverse the movement by coming up
again to the start position. Continue for desired reps.
**Do Not Bounce.**

# Chapter 9:

# LOWER BACK HAMSTRINGS

# DEVELOP POWERFUL LOWER BACK MUSCLES

## 09 DEVELOP POWERFUL LOWER-BACK MUSCLES

### POWERFUL LOWER BACK MUSCLES

**Develop Powerful Lower back muscles**

The lower back muscles support the lower part of the spine. When these muscles are well developed it builds a brace protecting the spine.

Apart from that the lower back muscles are responsible for bringing the body upright from a leaning forward position. Not only will the lower back be involved, but the glutes and hamstrings come into play as well.

## LOWER BACK EXERCISES

# 09 DEVELOP POWERFUL LOWER BACK/HAMSTRINGS

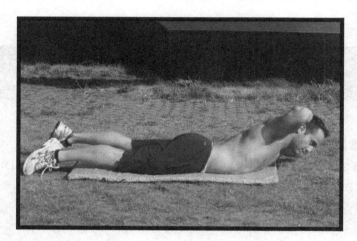

## LOWER BACK EXTENSION

As shown above this is the finished position. Lay flat on the floor and perform this movement by raising the upper body upwards slowly and pause for 2 seconds at the top. Reverse the movement slowly under control.

## LOWER BACK EXERCISES

## 09 DEVELOP POWERFUL LOWER BACK/HAMSTRINGS

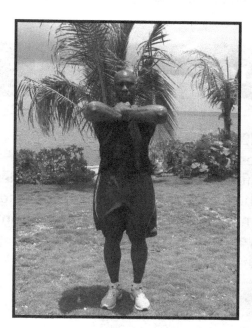
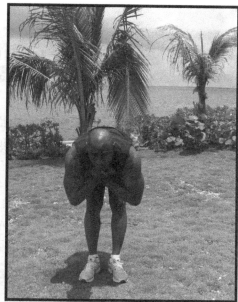

## STIFF LEGGED PRESS

Place the hands on your chest. Now press downwards while resisting with the hands until you are in the finished position. Relax and repeat for reps. This prestretches the hamstrings and adds strength to the lower back musculature.

# DEVELOP POWERFUL HAMSTRINGS

## 09 DEVELOP POWERFUL LOWER BACK/HAMSTRINGS

## DEVELOP STEEL CORD HAMSTRINGS

### DEVELOP STEEL CORD HAMSTRINGS

The hamstrings are the muscles at the back of the thighs.
These muscles are very powerful and work with the thigh muscles,
hips, glutes and lower-back. The hamstrings are taxed in sporting
activities, and although these muscles are not seen from the front
they are often neglected. However, with The Power Max
Transformation Method we have this covered.

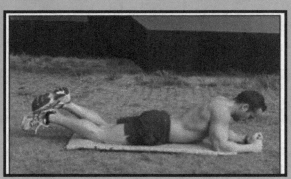

### HAMSTRING CURLS

While on the stomach on the floor place the left leg over the right as
shown, Now pull the right leg upwards towards you while resisting
with the left leg. Pull on the up phase only.

## LOWER BACK/HAMSTRING EXERCISES

## 09 DEVELOP POWERFUL LOWER BACK

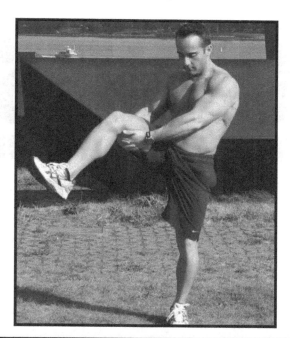

## THIGH ROWS

Interlock the fingers behind the knee as shown with right leg. With both arms pull the thigh upwards towards the chest while resisting with the leg. This exercise not only stimulate the upper back, it works the lowerback as well. Work one side fully then switch sides.

# Chapter 10:

# CALVES
## DEVELOP SHAPELY CALVES

# DEVELOP SHAPELY CALVES

## 10 DEVELOP SHAPELY CALVES

### DEVELOP SHAPELY CALVES

**Develop shapely calves**

The calves add a finished look to the lower leg with a diamond shape. This muscle has three heads (muscle parts) the soleus, this is under the large lateral head and gives the calves a full developed look viewed from the side and back.

The lateral and medial heads which are on the insides and in the middle of the muscle. The gastrocnemius make up the majority of the calf muscle. However, the longer the gastroc, the larger the potential for enhanced calf muscle development.

With The Power Max Transformation Method the stretch component adds strength, shape and muscle development quick.

## DEVELOP SHAPELY CALVES

# 10 DEVELOP SHAPELY CALVES

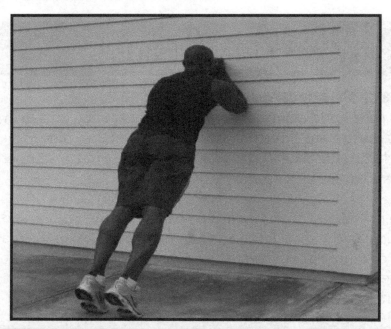

## SLANTED CALVE RAISES

Stand at least 30 inches away from the wall, or position yourself as shown but make sure the calves are well stretched. Start off as shown in the picture start position. Press straight up on the toes then lower. This is as awesome calve stretch exercise. Perform this exercise until the calves are well tired.
This stimulates the entire calve.

# Chapter 11:

# ABDOMINALS
## DEVELOP RIPPED ABS

# DEVELOP RIPPED ABS

## 11 DEVELOP RIPPED ABS

The abdominal muscles very important by revealing that the trainee has a lean physique. Plus the role of the abdominal muscles is to protect the spine. A lean chiseled set of abdominal muscles shows the opposite sex that the owner has a sign of virility.

Once these muscles are well developed this keeps the waist line and belly flat. There are various muscle structures that complete the overall look, the entire length of the abdominal wall, plus the internal and external obliques.

The lower sections of the abdominal muscles play the largest role in pro tecting the spine and storing belly fat. This is the easiest place for body fat to accumulate. Which makes training with self resistance the ideal exerciseto attack those muscle fibers to the maximum.

We cover the exercises that get the job done within this chapter.

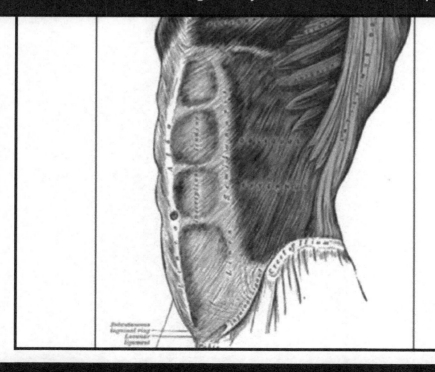

## DEVELOP RIPPED ABS

## 11 DEVELOP RIPPED ABS

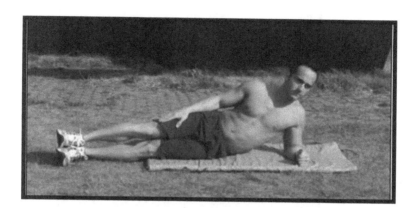

## DEVELOP RIPPED ABDOMINALS

As noted in the introduction the abdominal wall includes four muscles: Let's cover the front first, which is the entire length from the chest to pubis is called the rectus abdominis, people simply say abs for short. The abdominal wall should be worked in three angles of flexion. The lower sections of the abdominal muscles. The upper sections of the abdominal wall, and the obliques. Which are rotator muscles.

## DEVELOP RIPPED ABS

# 11 DEVELOP RIPPED ABS

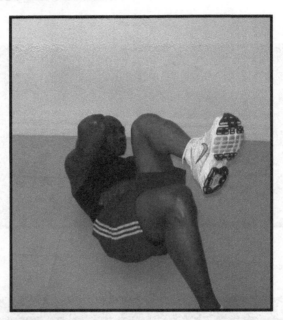

## ACROSS THE BODY OBLIQUE CRUNCH

Normally people say I want to lose my love handles.
Well rest assured this abdominal exercise really isolates the oblique muscles. These muscles supports the spine by making the abdominal wall more rigid.
Start off flat on the floor with right hand by the ear or behind the head. Knees together feet on floor, place the non-working arm on the floor or on the stomach. Now rotate towards the left knee as shown while bringing it towards the elbow.
While touching reverse the movement by going down lowering the foot in line with the other leg. Perform for reps then change sides.

## DEVELOP RIPPED ABS

# 11 DEVELOP RIPPED ABS

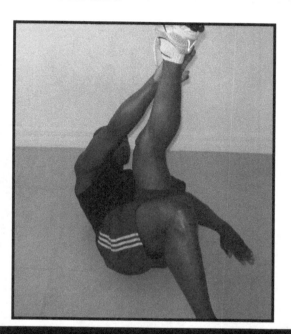

## ACROSS THE BODY OBLIQUE CRUNCH

Same exercise with a leg extension for variety

## DEVELOP RIPPED ABS

## 11 DEVELOP RIPPED ABS

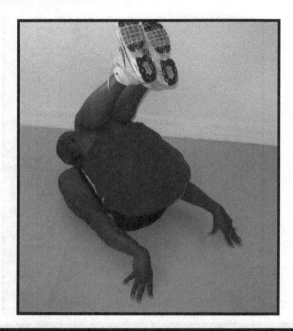

## REVERSE ABDOMINAL CRUNCHES

Start as shown roll the hip as you bring the knees into the chest and continue for desired reps.

# Chapter 12:

# ULTIMATE DENSITY METHOD
## DEVELOP POWERFUL MUSCLES FAST

## ULTIMATE DENSITY METHOD

# 12 ULTIMATE DENSITY METHOD

The Power Max Method is a slash between endurance-oriented fiber overload and a power element. It consists of various phases and multiple-reps, combined with a pause method that will increase your strength, muscle size and build muscle density. The reason for this, is that most trainees are not activating the endurance components of the fast-twitch 2A fibers.

The best part about The Power Max Method, is that it stimulates the mito-chondria in the muscle cells. Plus the noncontractile proteins that do not directly contribute to the production of muscle force. This will begin to produce new muscle-growth and strength gains at a **FASTER** rate.

The reason the Power Max Method works like a charm is the endurance component effect. Longer tension times, short rest between sets, and added fatigue accumulation. This form of training requires less force, but equals awesome hypertrophy pathways that build every facet of the muscle structure. So in short, you get larger muscles faster!

The Power Max Method have been tested on various subjects and it works **FAST**. Many would be skeptical with the high rep range at the start of the set. However, in truth, we do not need ultra-high resistance to grow. We have been brainwashed into thinking heavy weights is the only method to an awesome body. Not any more.

In truth, we have a massive amount of predominance type 2A power endur ance fibers. And the Power Max Method really stimulate and stress the sarcoplasm that gives the trainee a triple dose of increased muscle growth. The Power Max Method gets the job done in far less time. On top of that you will use various exercises to stimulate different fibers, this stimulate the bulk of the muscle for enhanced ongoing muscle-growth. Plus, muscle recruitment changes with each exercise and angle of pull.

**ULTIMATE DENSITY METHOD**

# 12 ULTIMATE DENSITY METHOD

We have the best exercises for enhancing muscle growth and strength for every body part. The Power Max exercises and methods provide continuous tension on the working muscles that increase growth producing fiber expansion.

How does the Power Max Method works in building larger muscles? It is a spectacular muscle-producing plan because you are cramming a lot of contractions into a short amount of time. By performing 20 reps, followed by 10 reps, then 5 reps with a 5 second break between each round of reps pre-fatiguing the fibers for more growth activation within the upcoming reps.

This muscle building method is a serious density producing formula. The method works because it targets the motor units to perform extensive repetitive work. This creates unwanted irritation on the muscles being worked, adaptation takes place where the muscles are forced to increase its size.

How do we perform The Power Max Method? Let's look at Phase one, using the bicep curl as an example.....Perform 20 reps, rest 5 seconds, perform another 10 reps, rest for another 5 seconds, then perform a final 5 reps. That's **ONE SET**. Then switch arms and repeat. This is a powerful muscle-producing-method and will really tax those 2A fast twitch endurance fibers to the max. Okay, so now you understand the concept, it is time to build some serious muscle with Phase one of The Power Max Method.

# 12 ULTIMATE DENSITY METHOD

This book is designed to enhance contractability within the muscle's structure in a safe approach by increasing time under-load with additional lactic acid buildup to enhance GH production levels once done long enough. The last thing the trainee will be doing is a work set allowing them 60 seconds of load time. This is not the best training model if the trainee is looking at significantly increasing muscle stimulation.

Most trainees need an extended period of 60 plus seconds of tension and load time if they want to coax muscle growth—for many trainees, this will be of great benefit with extended load times due to endurance-oriented fast-twitch-fibers. So, with The Power Max Method you get more intensity, longer load times, along with extensive fiber recruitment and muscle coaxing anabolic production. Another benefit that is extremely important is increased capillarization.

The Power Max Method will build more capillaries within the muscle struture, which in turn will give it more girth and make it more efficient at removing unwanted waste products while pushing growth nutrients within the muscle cell. The pump increases muscle growth, conditioning and strength levels, which is the best way to build an amazingly chiseled and healthy physique.

The amazing and exciting aspect about the self resistance exercises is that it will triple the speed at which you gain muscle and strength. This book clears up the confusion that exists when it comes to increasing muscle size and shape. Let's go over the massive myth which needs some expansion.
First off there is a direct correlation between muscle strength and size gains. With The Power Max Method while your strength increases you get bigger muscles, and will achieve powerful muscle growth allowing you reach your ultimate muscle and strength potential.

**ULTIMATE DENSITY METHOD**

# 12 ULTIMATE DENSITY METHOD

My promise is that you will build every hypertrophic constituent to where your physique will become shredded, with eye-popping carved out muscle at every limb—and it will not take years to reach that goal. Trainees that carry out training with The Power Max Method will acheive pumped up muscles like never before. The restriction of blood flow to the muscles with enhanced tension times is painful but it works like magic.

Alot of nitric oxide is released within the system, which will dilate blood vessels in an attempt to overcome the decreased blood flow within the muscle fibers, this however activates growth hormone release.

All the added force increases in the sarcoplasmic fluid as it builds new and more efficient energy substrates and mitochondria to supercompensate for the oxygen debt from the extended set protocol. Muscular development is mostly the result of blood blockage (occlusion) and sarcoplasmic growth from the isometric holds and extended continuous-tension force.

That is why The Power Max muscle-program was developed. Moderate intensity loads is best for muscle growth triggers, along with an increase and special focus on the force output approach on the exercises. Extended-load time training with (medium-high intensity) for an extended set protocol, with no real rest between exercises is best to coax the muscle-building effect.

Cutting rest time between exercises has a large impact on the growth of the musculature. Once you follow the exercise protocol in this book you do not allow your muscles to recover between exercises, which will coax the release of growth hormone prompting, greater muscle growth. So in short, training the muscle in a fatigued state—with extended tension with a high amount of work, is the most efficient way to build larger stronger muscles faster.

## ULTIMATE DENSITY METHOD

# 12 ULTIMATE DENSITY METHOD

This is why saraoplasmic wins due to the increase. However myofibrillar increases may be secondary here, but getting growth in the myofibrils will definetly add to a muscle's overall size. So, while sarcoplasmic increases is the primary growth factor in muscle tissue, it may be more true for some muscles than others.

Endurance-oriented muscle groups like forearms, abdominals, traps, hamstrings and calves respond best to sarcoplasmic stimulation in the majority of trainees. In most people, less-endurance-oriented muscle-groups require more of a balance of myofibrillar and sarcoplasmic stimulation to coax the greatest growth capacity. Nevertheless, with The Power Max Method you will be training both "sides" of the type-2A fibers to achieve maximum muscle stimulation. So it is the time under load that governs optimal muscle-building size stimulation.

Thats why The Power Max Method is so effective. Tension time is enhanced and this creates drastic sarcoplasm stress for size increases and cause fatigue components for myofibrillar power stimulation. In simple terms, an extended exercise set primarily activates sarcoplasmic expansion.
Which coax optimal size stimulation in both the myofibrils and sarcoplasm so you need to stimulate the two bases— tension/force for the myofibrils and extended load times for the sarcoplasm.

The extreme pump and burn indicates big sarcoplasmic-expansion effects. Thats why once the targeted muscle is under load for an extended period it will coax optimum sarcoplasmic stimulus, along with enhancing myofibrillar trauma and muscle-building growth activation. The bonus, is that the myofibrillar trauma also increases metabolic ramps that burns more bodyfat. So you will get more muscular and leaner at the same time! Now lets get some muscle-building going.

## 20,10,5 METHOD PHASE ONE

# 12 20,10,5 METHOD

### MONDAY, WEDNESDAY, FRIDAY (CHEST, BACK, MID-BACK, BICEPS, CALVES)

Perform each exercise with the 20,10, 5 method before moving to the next exercise. When the full cycle is completed, perform another round. Perform phase one for 2 weeks before moving to phase two.

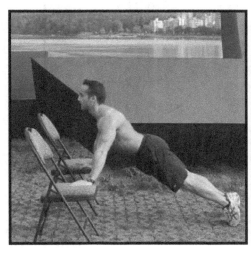
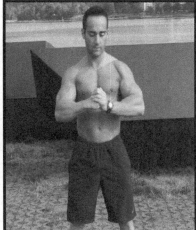
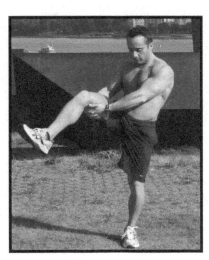
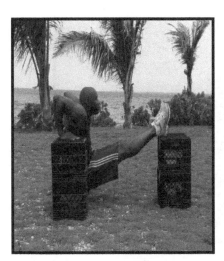

# 20,10,5   METHOD PHASE ONE

## 12   20,10, 5 METHOD

**MONDAY, WEDNESDAY, FRIDAY**
**Routine continued.........**

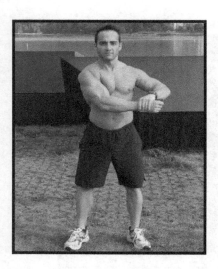
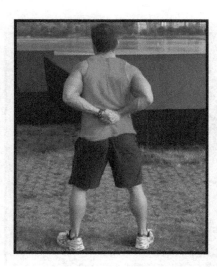
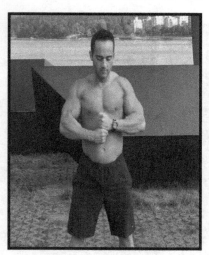
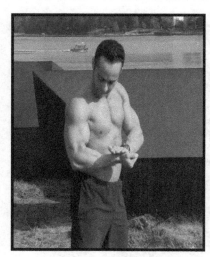

## 20,10,5  METHOD PHASE ONE

# 12 20,10,5 METHOD

**MONDAY, WEDNESDAY, FRIDAY**
**Routine continued...........**

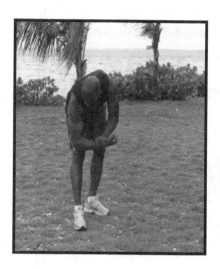 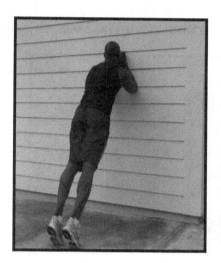

## PHASE ONE  MON, WED, FRI

# 20,10,5   METHOD PHASE ONE

## 12  20,10,5 METHOD

**TUESDAY, THURSDAY, SATURDAY (SHOULDERS, TRICEPS, THIGHS, HAMSTRINGS, ABS**
Perform each exercise with the 20/10/5 method before moving to the next exercise. When the full cycle is completed, perform another round. Perform phase one for 2 weeks before moving to phase two.

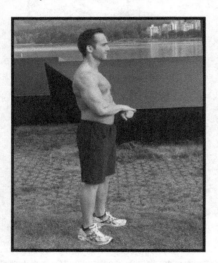
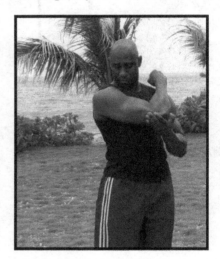
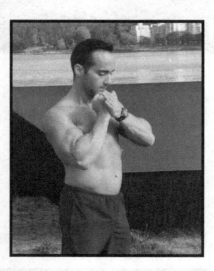
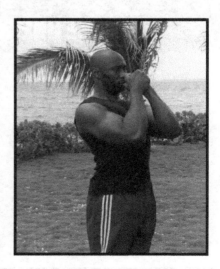

# 20,10,5  METHOD PHASE ONE

## 12  20,10,5 METHOD

**TUESDAY, THURSDAY, SATURDAY**
**Continued routine..........**

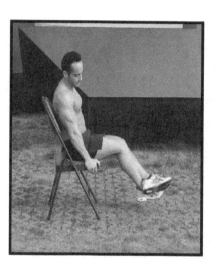
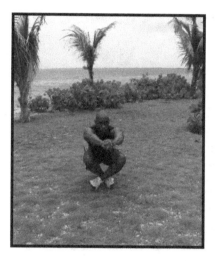

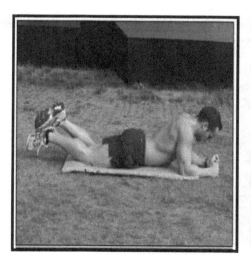
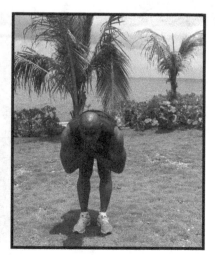

## 20,10,5  METHOD PHASE ONE

# 12  20,10,5 METHOD

**TUESDAY, THURSDAY, SATURDAY**
**Continued routine........**

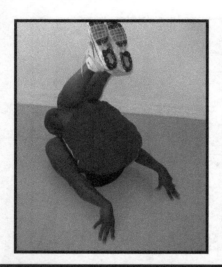
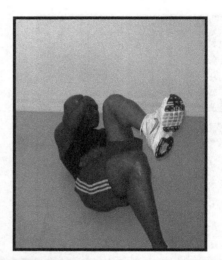

## PHASE ONE  TUES, THURS, SAT.

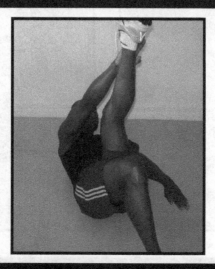

# PHASE TWO

## 13 MUSCLE BUILDING ACCELERATION PROGRAM

### MONDAY, WEDNESDAY, FRIDAY (BACK, ABS, LOWERBACK, CALVES, CHEST, SHOULDERS)

Within this phase perform the exercises on each page without rest until 3 rounds are completed. Perform 15 reps per exercise moving from exercise to exercise without rest. Perform this rotine for 2 weeks.

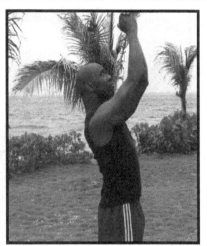
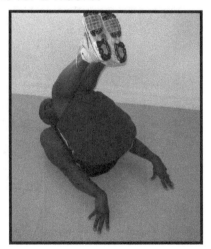
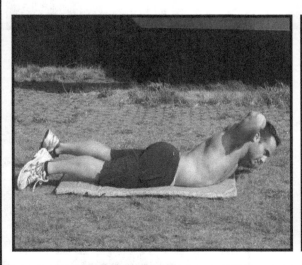
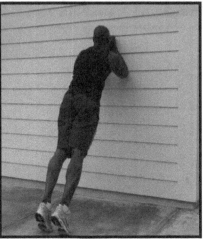

# PHASE TWO

## 13 MUSCLE BUILDING ACCELERATION PROGRAM

### MONDAY, WEDNESDAY, FRIDAY

Perform the exercises on this page non-stop until 3 rounds are completed.
Perform 15 reps per exercise.

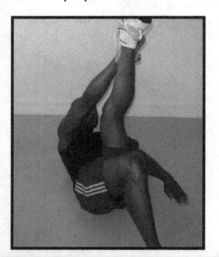

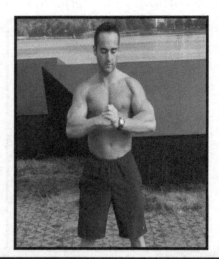

## PHASE TWO   MON, WED, FRI.

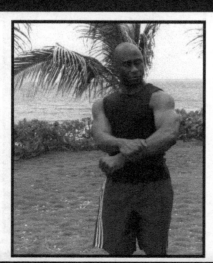

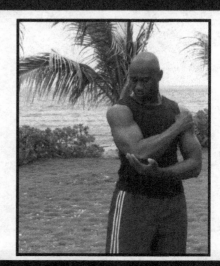

# PHASE TWO

## 13 MUSCLE BUILDING ACCELERATION PROGRAM

**TUESDAY, THURSDAY, SATURDAY (MID-BACK, BACK, BICEPS, TRICEPS, BACK, ABS)**
Perform the exercises on this page non-stop until 3 rounds are completed.
Perform 15 reps per exercise.

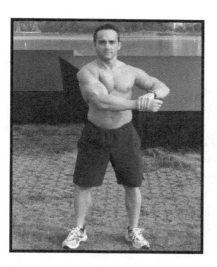
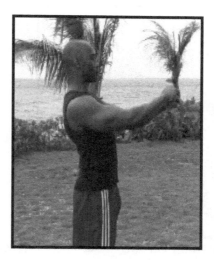

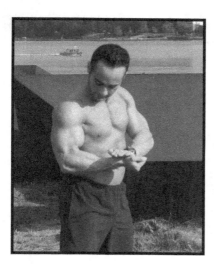
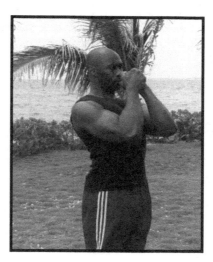

# PHASE TWO

## 13 MUSCLE BUILDING ACCELERATION PROGRAM

**TUESDAY, THURSDAY, SATURDAY**
Perform the exercises on this page non-stop until 3 rounds are completed. Perform 15 reps per exercise.

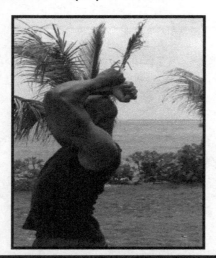
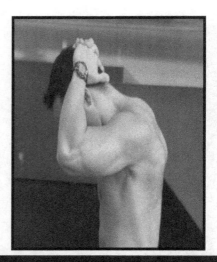

## PHASE TWO   TUES, THURS, SAT.

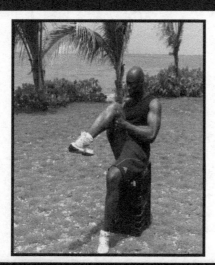
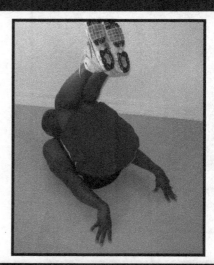

# ENHANCING MUSCLE FIBER ACTIVATION

## 14 MUSCLE BUILDING ACCELERATION PROGRAM

### Enhancing-Muscle-Fiber-Activation

The first thing The Power Max Method will address is the understanding of how to irritate and coax muscle growth and strength with the Muscle-Building-Module of muscle-fiber-stimulation.

**Type 1s** Are aerobic, and require oxygen to fire, it contains loads of mitochondria, where fat is burned for energy. With our program you will call on these fibers a lot!

**Type 2As** Have both aerobic and anaerobic components. You will use these for low-contraction isometric work. Mitochondria is present, but far fewer than the type 1s.

In all truth, these fiber types fire on a multi-extending set principle, but at different capacities. So, the harder the contraction, the less your type1s come into play. So on extreme force with strength-building self resistance contractions, (which I do not recommend) very few type 1s fire; however, ultra-heavy isometric contractions is not the best way to create and coax muscle size and strength gains. The reason...

The trainee need increased time under load to coax the muscle fibers to grow, so in truth trainees need to emphasize the endurance-fast-twitch-fibers to increase muscle size and strength. So if you're looking for increased muscle growth, medium intensity contractions will get the job done safely and effectively.

By combining the various tension times within the pages of The Power Max Method you will train all facets of the muscle for optimal development and strength. This book shows you how to perform these simple and unique exercises safely and effectively, by increasing the (myofibrils) and the more endurance part (sarcoplasm), not to mention the type-1 aerobic fibers.

# ENHANCING MUSCLE FIBER ACTIVATION

## 14 MUSCLE BUILDING ACCELERATION PROGRAM

### Enhancing-Muscle-Fiber-Activation

It has been suggested that Isometrics need to be performed at high intensities for low second holds that proclaim is the key to optimum muscle growth and strength. That is not 100 percent accurate; you see, most recommend trainees perform a 5-10 second isometric static hold. If they do this, the target muscle is only under tension for a short time. This is not an effective way to get ripped, increase muscle size or maintain healthy joints, by using that time under load frame, lots of sarcoplasmic "endurance" growth potential effects are left out.

You want both medium and longer tension times for optimum muscle-building stimulation, which can be achieved with various contractions in the 30 to 40 second range, or tension that last up to 60-plus seconds, for 2A sarcoplasmic expansion + endurance power type-1 activation along with safe tendon strengthening.

Using the methods within these pages with moderate tension will build up more muscle strength with healthy tendons, than people that train in the traditional way of high resistance. Performing the contractions with moderate resistance will result in leaner, stronger and bigger muscles for life..

The reason being, with moderate tension sets the trainee can fatigue the endurance slow-twitch fibers, with more precision at the beginning of the extended set. This forces more endurance fast-twitch fibers to fire after 40 plus seconds, exactly what you need to coax more muscle. Okay, so now you under stand the extended set muscle enhancing method.

# ENHANCING MUSCLE FIBER ACTIVATION

## 14 MUSCLE BUILDING ACCELERATION PROGRAM

### The "Extended Power Pump" extention for Quality Muscle

What is the ideal time under tension isometric hold for increasing sculpted muscle-gains? In all truth, doing sets with 20 plus extended holds in a few phases gets the muscle-building job done. It's a special blow-torch Isometric Power phase which, will produce increased hardening and will induce the fat-burning process along with increasing an amazing pump to coax muscle-building-gains.

Now why is it by doing extended-endurance-type isometric holds build lean muscle and increases strength gains more effectively? Because, it causes more intense contractions to the targeted muscle fibers more times over than so-called "traditional" isometric holds, this increases greater degrees of protein remodeling in the targeted muscles.

So in other words, the extended tension times cause more muscle irritation, which activates significantly more endurance-fast-twitch power fibers. We are lead to believe that intense powerful isometric holds of 5-10 seconds will yeild the best gains—NO. Doing high tension isometric holds will lead to tendon damage and muscle strain.

# ENHANCING MUSCLE FIBER ACTIVATION

## 14 MUSCLE BUILDING ACCELERATION PROGRAM

### What is a Self-resistance-Isometric contraction

An Isometric contraction is where the trainee apply force and hold that contraction by maintaining a static position. This increases tension (force out put) on the muscle fibers to promote muscular tension which produce strength gains.

A classic example is shown in the picture below by placing the hands at chest level and pressing the palms together holding the contraction for seconds at a time. Please note while performing all of the Isometric exercises it is important that you breathe normally. **DO NOT HOLD YOUR BREATH**

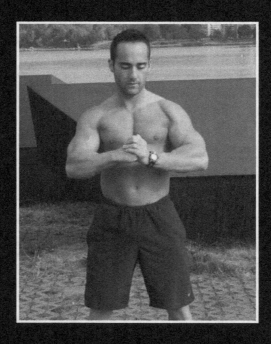

# Chapter 14:

# ENHANCING MUSCLE FIBER ACTIVATION
## MUSCLE ACCELERATION PROGRAMS

# ENHANCING MUSCLE FIBER ACTIVATION

## 14 MUSCLE ACCELERATION PROGRAM

### HOW TO PERFORM THIS ROUTINE:

Perform 15 reps in total. On your 11th rep perform an isometric contraction at the contracted position for 5 seconds on each of the 5 reps. Until you have completed 15 reps for that set. Perform 15 reps at 3 sets each exercise. Resting 10 seconds between sets. Perform this program for 2 weeks.

**DAY ONE**

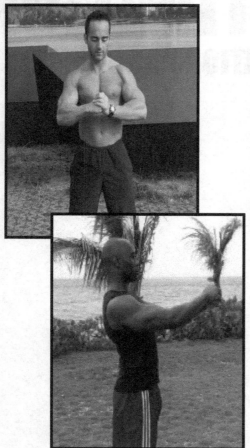
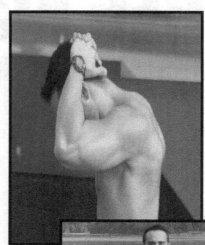
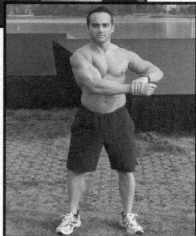

# ENHANCING MUSCLE FIBER ACTIVATION

## 14  MUSCLE ACCELERATION PROGRAM

### HOW TO PERFORM THIS ROUTINE:

Perform 15 reps in total. On your 11th rep perform an isometric contraction at the contracted position for 5 seconds on each of the 5 reps. Until you have completed 15 reps for that set. Perform 15 reps at 3 sets each exercise. Resting 10 seconds between sets.

### DAY ONE continued..........

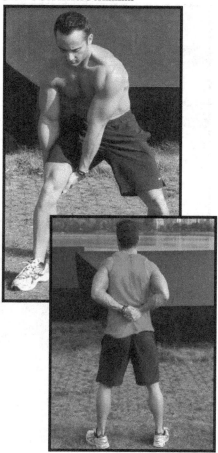

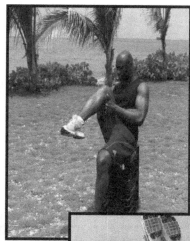

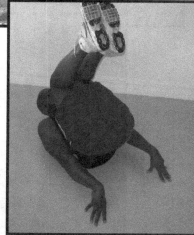

# ENHANCING MUSCLE FIBER ACTIVATION

## 14 MUSCLE ACCELERATION PROGRAM

### HOW TO PERFORM THIS ROUTINE:

Perform 15 reps in total. On your 11th rep perform an isometric contraction at the contracted position for 5 seconds on each of the 5 reps. Until you have completed 15 reps for that set. Perform 15 reps at 3 sets each exercise. Resting 10 seconds between sets.

**DAY TWO**

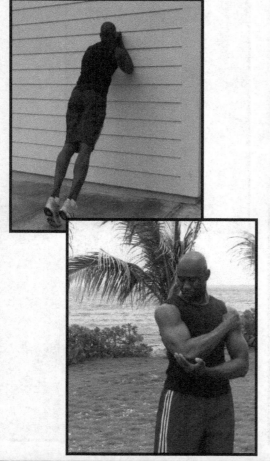
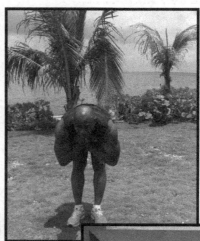
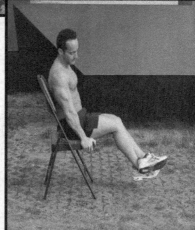

# ENHANCING MUSCLE FIBER ACTIVATION

## 14 MUSCLE ACCELERATION PROGRAM

### HOW TO PERFORM THIS ROUTINE:

Perform 15 reps in total. On your 11th rep perform an isometric contraction at the contracted position for 5 seconds on each of the 5 reps. Until you have completed 15 reps for that set. Perform 15 reps at 3 sets each exercise. Resting 10 seconds between sets.

### DAY TWO continued.............

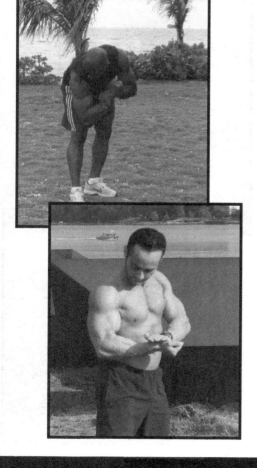
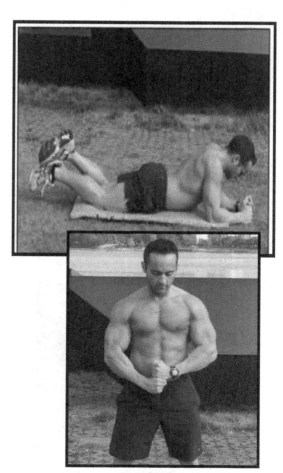

# ENHANCING MUSCLE FIBER ACTIVATION

## 14 MUSCLE ACCELERATION PROGRAM

### HOW TO PERFORM THIS ROUTINE:

Perform 15 reps in total. On your 11th rep perform an isometric contraction at the contracted position for 5 seconds on each of the 5 reps. Until you have completed 15 reps for that set. Perform 15 reps at 3 sets each exercise. Resting 10 seconds between sets.

### DAY THREE

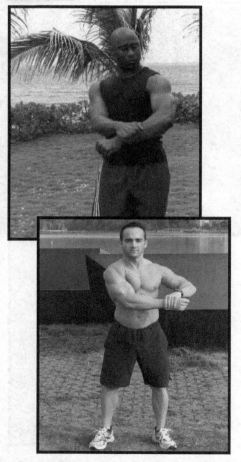

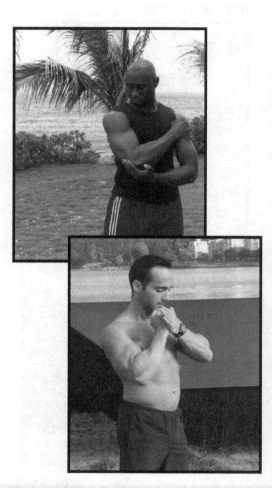

# ENHANCING MUSCLE FIBER ACTIVATION

## 14 MUSCLE ACCELERATION PROGRAM

### HOW TO PERFORM THIS ROUTINE:

Perform 15 reps in total. On your 11th rep perform an isometric contraction at the contracted position for 5 seconds on each of the 5 reps. Until you have completed 15 reps for that set. Perform 15 reps at 3 sets each exercise. Resting 10 seconds between sets.

### DAY THREE continued.......

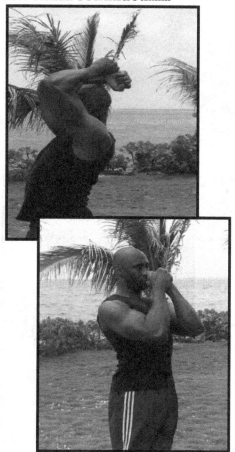

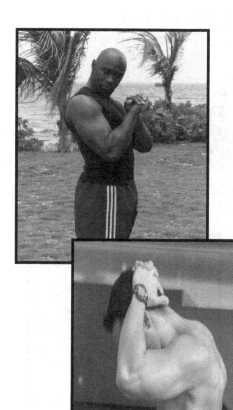

# ENHANCING MUSCLE FIBER ACTIVATION

## 14 MUSCLE ACCELERATION PROGRAM

### HOW TO PERFORM THIS ROUTINE:

Perform 15 reps in total. On your 11th rep perform an isometric contraction at the contracted position for 5 seconds on each of the 5 reps. Until you have completed 15 reps for that set. Perform 15 reps at 3 sets each exercise. Resting 10 seconds between sets.

**DAY THREE continued.......**

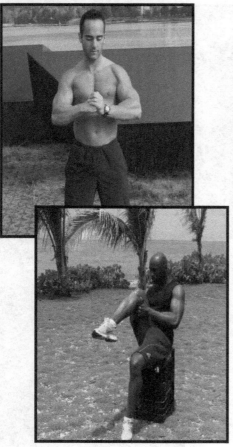
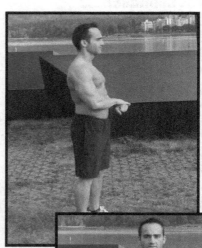
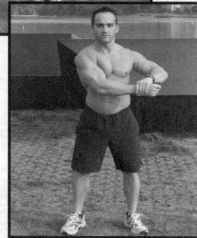

# ENHANCING MUSCLE FIBER ACTIVATION

## 14 MUSCLE ACCELERATION PROGRAM

### HOW TO PERFORM THIS ROUTINE:

Perform 15 reps in total. On your 11th rep perform an isometric contraction at the contracted position for 5 seconds on each of the 5 reps. Until you have completed 15 reps for that set. Perform 15 reps at 3 sets each exercise. Resting 10 seconds between sets.

### DAY FOUR

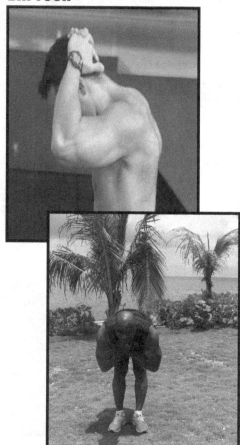

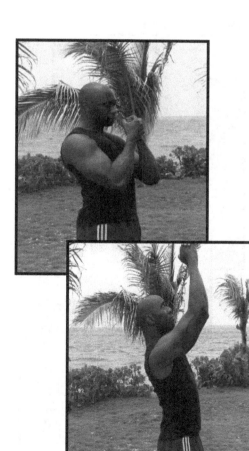

# ENHANCING MUSCLE FIBER ACTIVATION

## 14 MUSCLE ACCELERATION PROGRAM

### HOW TO PERFORM THIS ROUTINE:

Perform 15 reps in total. On your 11th rep perform an isometric contraction at the contracted position for 5 seconds on each of the 5 reps. Until you have completed 15 reps for that set. Perform 15 reps at 3 sets each exercise. Resting 10 seconds between sets.

**DAY FOUR continued......**

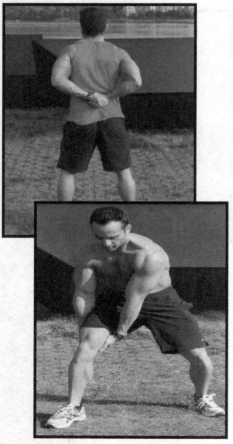

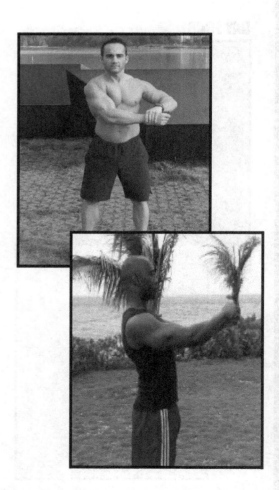

## ENHANCING MUSCLE FIBER ACTIVATION

# 14 MUSCLE ACCELERATION PROGRAM

### HOW TO PERFORM THIS ROUTINE:

Perform 15 reps in total. On your 11th rep perform an isometric contraction at the contracted position for 5 seconds on each of the 5 reps. Until you have completed 15 reps for that set. Perform 15 reps at 3 sets each exercise. Resting 10 seconds between sets.

### DAY FIVE

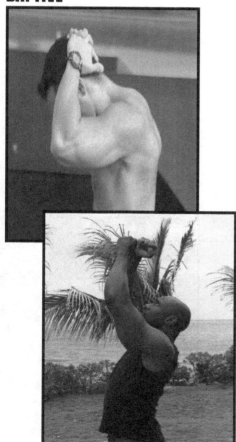

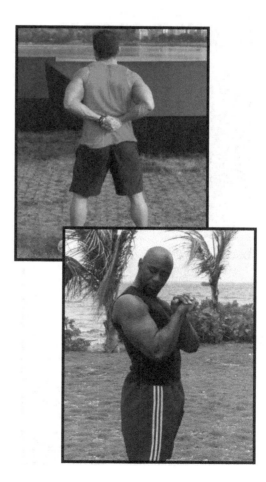

# ENHANCING MUSCLE FIBER ACTIVATION

## 14  MUSCLE ACCELERATION PROGRAM

### HOW TO PERFORM THIS ROUTINE:

Perform 15 reps in total. On your 11th rep perform an isometric contraction at the contracted position for 5 seconds on each of the 5 reps. Until you have completed 15 reps for that set.  Perform 15 reps at 3 sets each exercise. Resting 10 seconds between sets.

**DAY FIVE continued.....**

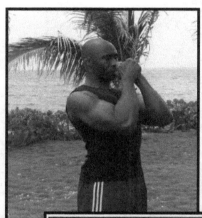

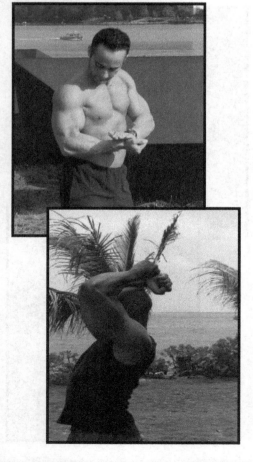

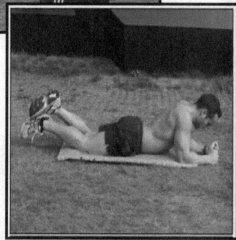

# THE ISOMETRIC POWER MAX PROGRAM PHASE ONE

# THE ISOMETRIC POWER MAX PROGRAM

## 15 THE ISOMETRIC POWER MAX PROGRAM

### ISOMETRIC POWER MAX PROGRAM "GET BIG PHASE"

**Phase 1:** Is the speed phase —you crank out as many 1 second reps as you can, at 20 reps per set. This faster cadence activates higher percentages of fast-twitch fibers, so it is one of the best growth-fiber-activating phases.

**Phase 2:** Is the power phase—you contract within 1 second and slowly release the tension for 3 seconds. This fatigues those last remaining fast-twitch fibers, pushing the muscle fibers past the growth threshold.

**Phase 3:** Is the strength phase—you contract for 2 seconds and release for a slow 6 seconds. This increases the muscle damage by increasing strength levels and growth hormone release due to the burning effect.

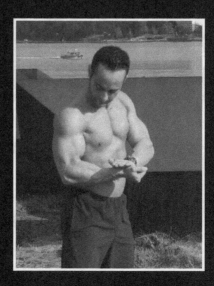

## THE ISOMETRIC POWER MAX PROGRAM

## 15 THE ISOMETRIC POWER MAX PROGRAM

### HOW TO PERFORM THIS ROUTINE:
### PHASE ONE SPEED PHASE

Perform the speed reps at 1 second contracted, 1 second release. Perform 20 reps per set with a 20 second isometric hold on the 20th rep.

**DAY ONE**

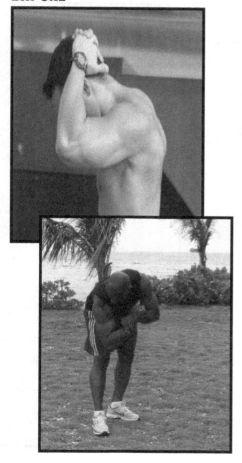

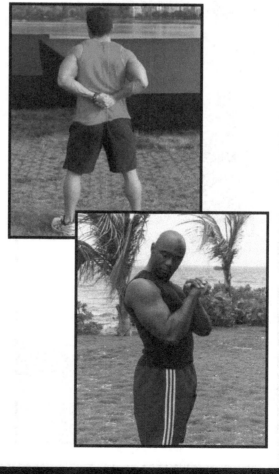

# THE ISOMETRIC POWER MAX PROGRAM

## 15 THE ISOMETRIC POWER MAX PROGRAM

### HOW TO PERFORM THIS ROUTINE:
### PHASE ONE SPEED PHASE

Perform the speed reps at 1 second contracted, 1 second release. Perform 20 reps per set with a 30 second isometric hold on the 20th rep.

**DAY ONE continued.............**

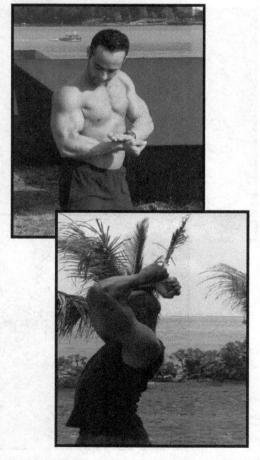

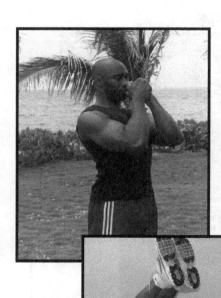

# THE ISOMETRIC POWER MAX PROGRAM

## 15 THE ISOMETRIC POWER MAX PROGRAM

### HOW TO PERFORM THIS ROUTINE:
### PHASE ONE SPEED PHASE

Perform the speed reps at 1 second contracted, 1 second release. Perform 20 reps per set with a 30 second isometric hold on the 20th rep.

### DAY TWO

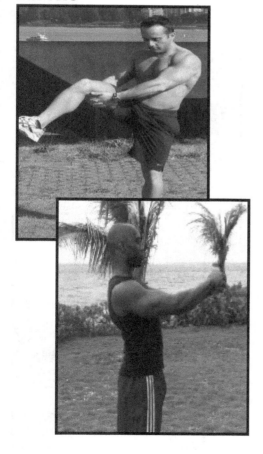

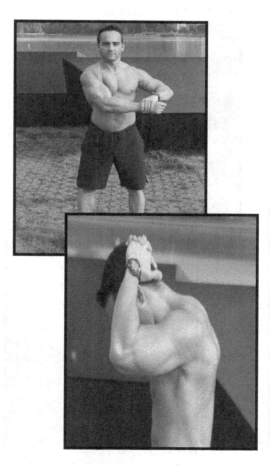

# THE ISOMETRIC POWER MAX PROGRAM

## 15 THE ISOMETRIC POWER MAX PROGRAM

### HOW TO PERFORM THIS ROUTINE:
### PHASE ONE SPEED PHASE

Perform the speed reps at 1 second contracted, 1 second release. Perform 20 reps per set with a 30 second isometric hold on the 20th rep.

**DAY TWO continued.......**

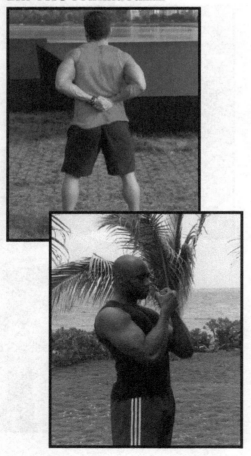
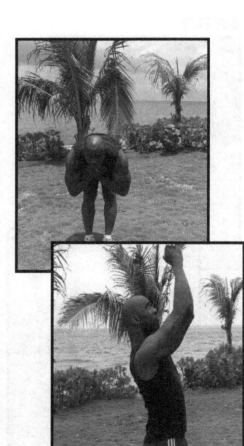

# THE ISOMETRIC POWER MAX PROGRAM

## 15 THE ISOMETRIC POWER MAX PROGRAM

### HOW TO PERFORM THIS ROUTINE:
### PHASE ONE SPEED PHASE

Perform the speed reps at 1 second contracted, 1 second release. Perform 20 reps per set with a 30 second isometric hold on the 20th rep.

### DAY THREE

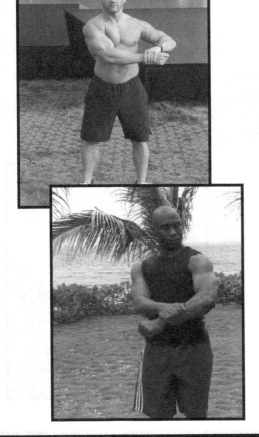
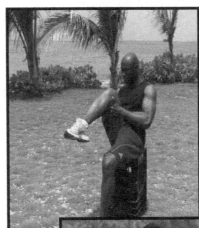
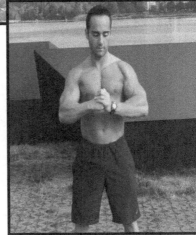

# THE ISOMETRIC POWER MAX PROGRAM

## 15  THE ISOMETRIC POWER MAX PROGRAM

### HOW TO PERFORM THIS ROUTINE:
### PHASE ONE SPEED PHASE

Perform the speed reps at 1 second contracted, 1 second release. Perform 20 reps per set with a 30 second isometric hold on the 20th rep.

**DAY THREE  continued.........**

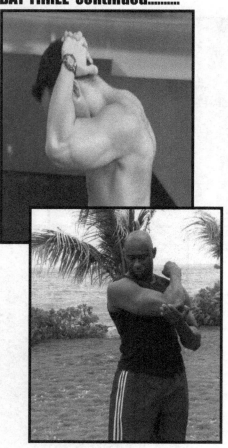

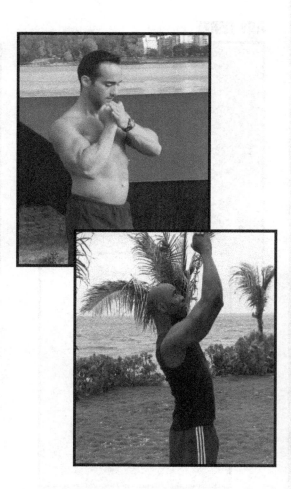

# THE ISOMETRIC POWER MAX PROGRAM

## 15 THE ISOMETRIC POWER MAX PROGRAM

### HOW TO PERFORM THIS ROUTINE:
### PHASE ONE SPEED PHASE

Perform the speed reps at 1 second contracted, 1 second release. Perform 20 reps per set with a 30 second isometric hold on the 20th rep.

**DAY FOUR**

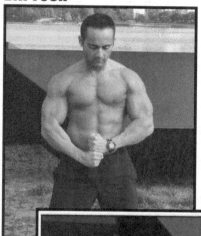
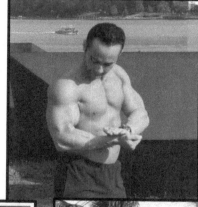
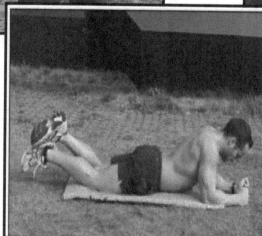
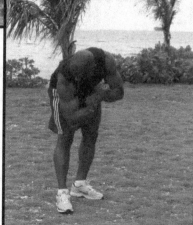

# THE ISOMETRIC POWER MAX PROGRAM

## 15 THE ISOMETRIC POWER MAX PROGRAM

### HOW TO PERFORM THIS ROUTINE:
### PHASE ONE SPEED PHASE

Perform the speed reps at 1 second contracted, 1 second release. Perform 20 reps per set with a 30 second isometric hold on the 20th rep.

**DAY FOUR continued...........**

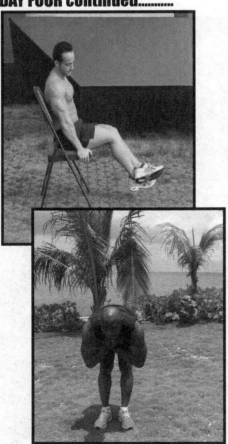

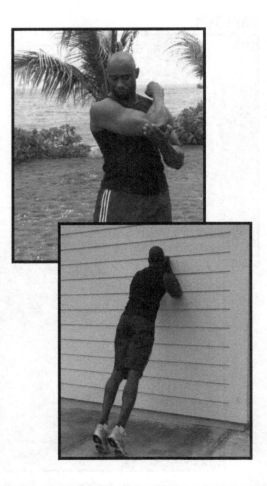

# THE ISOMETRIC POWER MAX PROGRAM

## 15 THE ISOMETRIC POWER MAX PROGRAM

### HOW TO PERFORM THIS ROUTINE:
### PHASE ONE  SPEED PHASE

Perform the speed reps at 1 second contracted, 1 second release. Perform 20 reps per set with a 30 second isometric hold on the 20th rep.

### DAY FIVE

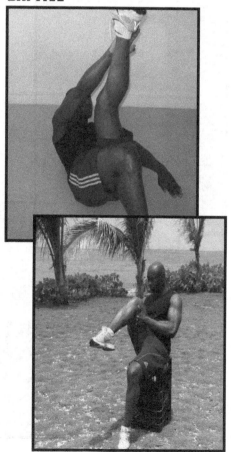

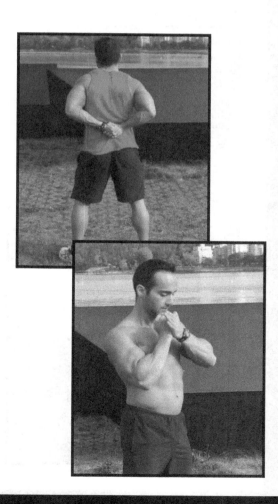

# THE ISOMETRIC POWER MAX PROGRAM

## 15 THE ISOMETRIC POWER MAX PROGRAM

### HOW TO PERFORM THIS ROUTINE:
### PHASE ONE SPEED PHASE

Perform the speed reps at 1 second contracted, 1 second release. Perform 20 reps per set with a 30 second isometric hold on the 20th rep.

**DAY FIVE continued............**

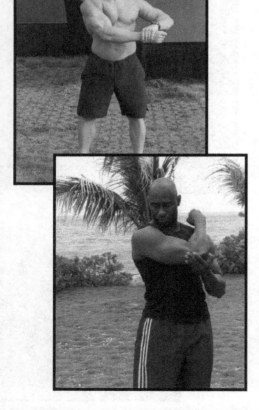

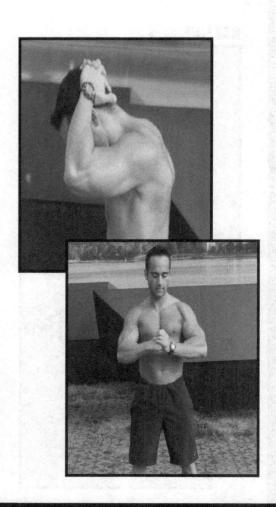

# THE ISOMETRIC POWER MAX PROGRAM PHASE TWO

# THE ISOMETRIC POWER MAX PROGRAM

## 15 THE ISOMETRIC POWER MAX PROGRAM

### HOW TO PERFORM THIS ROUTINE:
### PHASE TWO POWER PHASE

Perform the power phase—by contracting within 1 second then slowly reverse the movement for 3 seconds. Perform 7 reps. On the 7th perform a isometric hold for 10 seconds. Alternate day one and day two for 6 days per week of training. Perform this program for 2 weeks.

**DAY ONE**

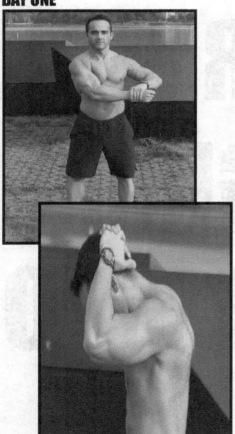

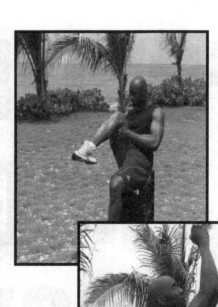

# THE ISOMETRIC POWER MAX PROGRAM

## 15 THE ISOMETRIC POWER MAX PROGRAM

### HOW TO PERFORM THIS ROUTINE:
### PHASE TWO POWER PHASE

Perform the power phase—by contracting within 1 second then slowly reverse the movement for 3 seconds. Perform 7 reps. On the 7th perform a isometric hold for 10 seconds. Alternate day one and day two for 6 days per week of training.

### DAY ONE continued..........

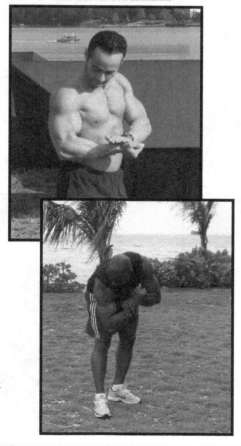

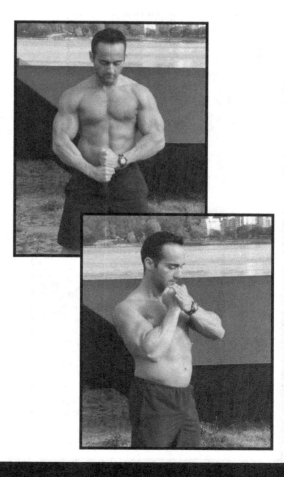

# THE ISOMETRIC POWER MAX PROGRAM

## 15 THE ISOMETRIC POWER MAX PROGRAM

### HOW TO PERFORM THIS ROUTINE:
### PHASE TWO POWER PHASE

Perform the power phase—by contracting within 1 second then slowly reverse the movement for 3 seconds. Perform 7 reps. On the 7th perform a isometric hold for 10 seconds. Alternate day one and day two for 6 days per week of training.

**DAY TWO**

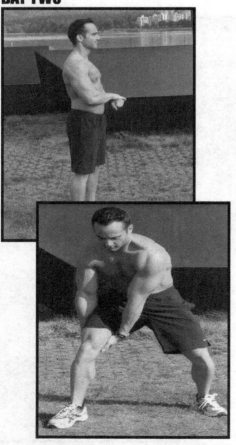

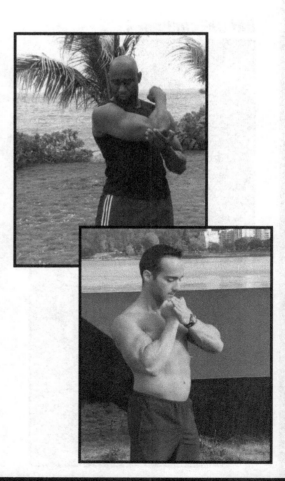

# THE ISOMETRIC POWER METHOD PROGRAM

## 15  THE ISOMETRIC POWER METHOD PROGRAM

### HOW TO PERFORM THIS ROUTINE:
### PHASE TWO POWER PHASE

Perform the power phase—by contracting within 1 second and slowly release the tension for 3 seconds. Perform 7 reps. On the 7th perform a isometric hold for 10 seconds. Alternate day one and day two for 6 days per week of training.

### DAY TWO continued........

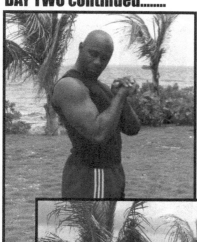

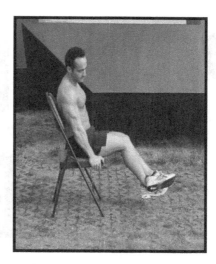

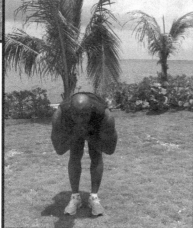

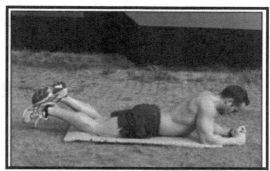

# Chapter 15:

# THE ISOMETRIC POWER MAX PROGRAM PHASE THREE

# THE ISOMETRIC POWER MAX PROGRAM

## 15 THE ISOMETRIC POWER MAX PROGRAM

### HOW TO PERFORM THIS ROUTINE:
### PHASE THREE STRENGTH PHASE

Perform this strength phase—by contracting for 2 seconds and release for a slow 6 seconds. On the 10th rep perform a 20 second isometric hold. This increases the muscle damage increasing strength levels and growth hormone release. Alternate day one and day two for 6 days per week.

### DAY ONE

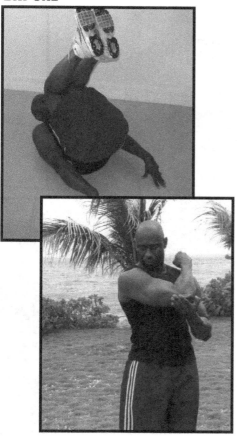

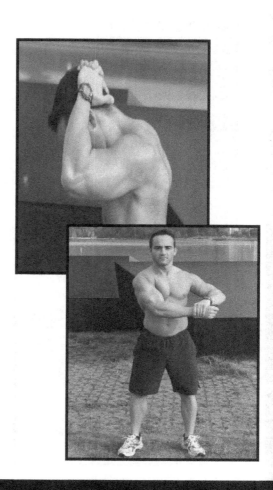

# THE ISOMETRIC POWER MAX PROGRAM

## 15 THE ISOMETRIC POWER MAX PROGRAM

### HOW TO PERFORM THIS ROUTINE:
### PHASE THREE STRENGTH PHASE

Perform this strength phase—by contracting for 2 seconds and release for a slow 6 seconds. On the 10th rep perform a 20 second isometric hold. This increases the muscle damage increasing strength levels and growth hormone release. Alternate day one and day two for 6 days per week.

**DAY ONE continued...........**

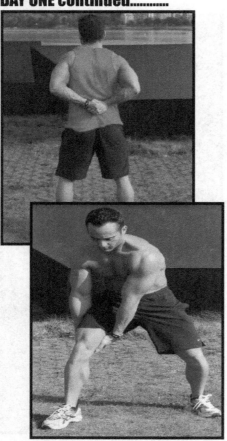

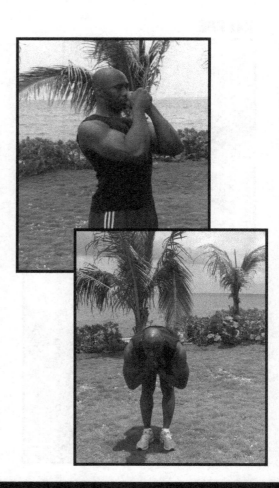

# THE ISOMETRIC POWER MAX PROGRAM

## 15  THE ISOMETRIC POWER MAX PROGRAM

### HOW TO PERFORM THIS ROUTINE:
### PHASE THREE STRENGTH PHASE

Perform this strength phase—by contracting for 2 seconds and release for a slow 6 seconds. On the 10th rep perform a 20 second isometric hold. This increases the muscle damage increasing strength levels and growth hormone release. Alternate day one and day two for 6 days per week.

**DAY TWO**

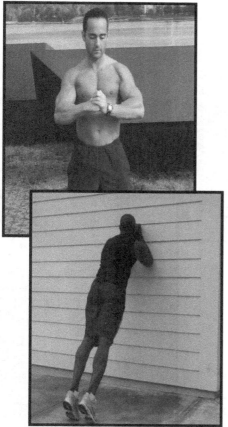

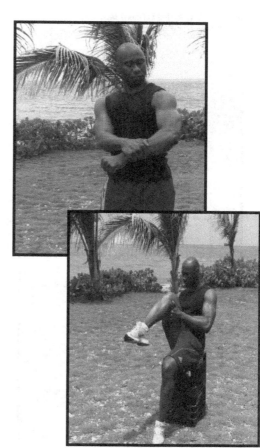

# THE ISOMETRIC POWER MAX PROGRAM

## 15 THE ISOMETRIC POWER MAX PROGRAM

### HOW TO PERFORM THIS ROUTINE:
### PHASE THREE STRENGTH PHASE

Perform this strength phase—by contracting for 2 seconds and release for a slow 6 seconds. On the 10th rep perform a 20 second isometric hold. This increases the muscle damage increasing strength levels and growth hormone release. Alternate day one and day two for 6 days per week.

**DAY TWO continued..........**

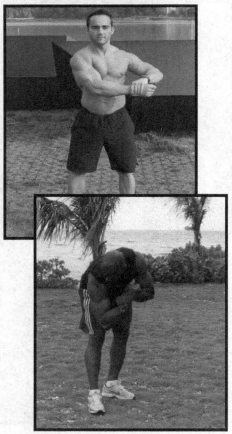

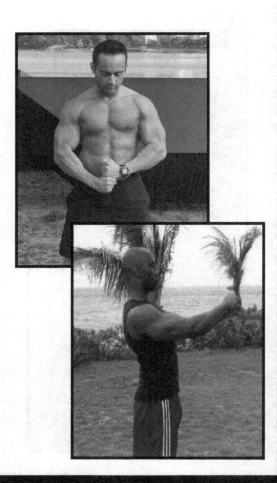

# Chapter 16

# THE ISOMETRIC 10,10,10 PROGRAM

# THE ISOMETRIC 10,10,10 PROGRAM

## 16  THE ISOMETRIC 10,10,10 PROGRAM

### THE ISOMETRIC 10/10/10 PROGRAM

The Power Max Transformation Method is a great multi-angular strength-enhancing system. Below is a great program The Isometric 10,10,10 Program. This is were you hammer your muscles non-stop for an intense fat burning trigger. How does this program burn bodyfat and increase lean muscle size?

As a result of these routines, in short, the trainee will move quickly from exercise to exercise with no rest between exercises to highten extreme fiber stimulation and increase fat-burning-hormonal release. Which is a fiber-activation growth enhancer. This method of extended-time under load sets coax additional growth fibers to fire rapidly within the contraction being held.

Below The Isometric 10,10,10 Program for each target muscle will host exercises to stimulate full Flexion and contractability. However the trainee will receive maximum muscle fiber and tendon stimulation with this Isometric Program.

# THE ISOMETRIC 10,10,10 PROGRAM

## 16  THE ISOMETRIC 10,10,10 PROGRAM

### HOW TO PERFORM THIS ROUTINE:
### THE ISOMETRIC FAT LOSS PROGRAM

Perform this **ISOMETRIC WORKOUT**—by placing the muscle at the mid-point contracted position. Hold that contracted position for 10,10,10 seconds each before moving onto another contraction. Perform all exercises one after the other until all exercises are completed without rest.  Perform 3 rounds of these between each round rest for 10 seconds before starting the round again.

**Alternate day one and day two for 6 days per week.**

**DAY ONE**

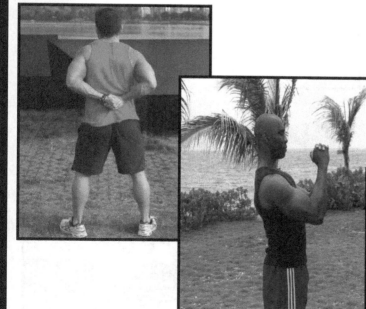

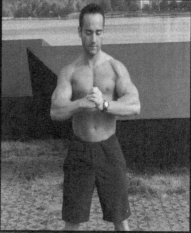

# THE ISOMETRIC 10,10,10 PROGRAM

## 16  THE ISOMETRIC 10,10,10 PROGRAM

### HOW TO PERFORM THIS ROUTINE:
### THE ISOMETRIC FAT LOSS PROGRAM

Perform this **ISOMETRIC WORKOUT**—by placing the muscle at the mid-point contracted position. Hold that contracted position for 10,10,10 seconds each before moving onto another contraction. Perform all exercises one after the other until all exercises are completed without rest.  Perform 3 rounds of these between each round rest for 10 seconds before starting the round again.
**Alternate day one and day two for 6 days per week.**
**DAY ONE continued.........**

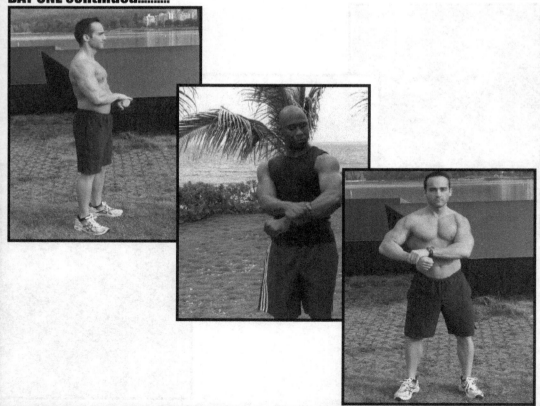

# THE ISOMETRIC 10,10,10 PROGRAM

## 16  THE ISOMETRIC 10,10,10 PROGRAM

**HOW TO PERFORM THIS ROUTINE:**
**THE ISOMETRIC FAT LOSS PROGRAM**

Perform this **ISOMETRIC WORKOUT**—by placing the muscle at the mid-point contracted position. Hold that contracted position for 10,10,10 seconds each before moving onto another contraction. Perform all exercises one after the other until all exercises are completed without rest.  Perform 3 rounds of these between each round rest for 10 seconds before starting the round again.
**Alternate day one and day two for 6 days per week.**
**DAY ONE continued......**

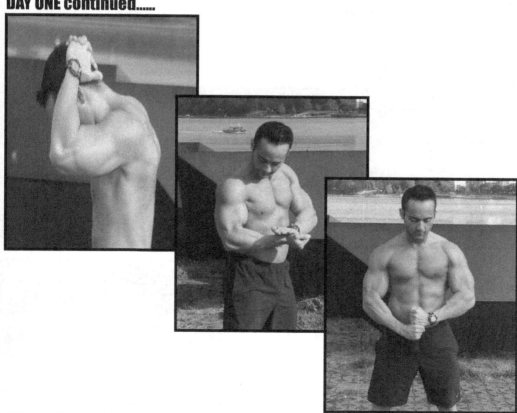

# THE ISOMETRIC 10,10,10 PROGRAM

## 16 THE ISOMETRIC 10,10,10 PROGRAM

### HOW TO PERFORM THIS ROUTINE:
### THE ISOMETRIC FAT LOSS PROGRAM

Perform this **ISOMETRIC WORKOUT**—by placing the muscle at the mid-point contracted position. Hold that contracted position for 10,10,10 seconds each before moving onto another contraction. Perform all exercises one after the other until all exercises are completed without rest. Perform 3 rounds of these between each round rest for 10 seconds before starting the round again.

**Alternate day one and day two for 6 days per week.**
**DAY TWO**

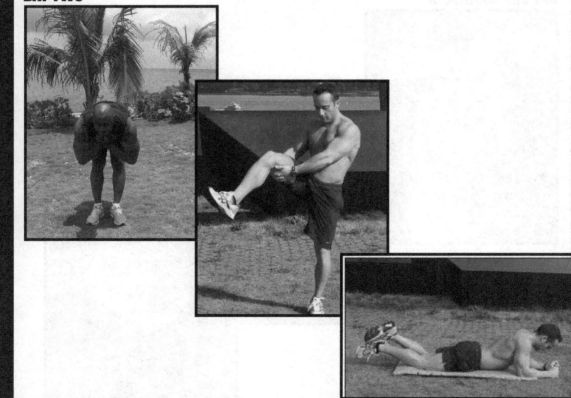

# THE ISOMETRIC 10,10,10 PROGRAM

## 16  THE ISOMETRIC 10,10,10 PROGRAM

### HOW TO PERFORM THIS ROUTINE:
### THE ISOMETRIC FAT LOSS PROGRAM

Perform this **ISOMETRIC WORKOUT**—by placing the muscle at the mid-point contracted position. Hold that contracted position for 10,10,10 seconds each before moving onto another contraction. Perform all exercises one after the other until all exercises are completed without rest.  Perform 3 rounds of these between each round rest for 10 seconds before starting the round again.

**Alternate day one and day two for 6 days per week.**
**DAY TWO continue........**

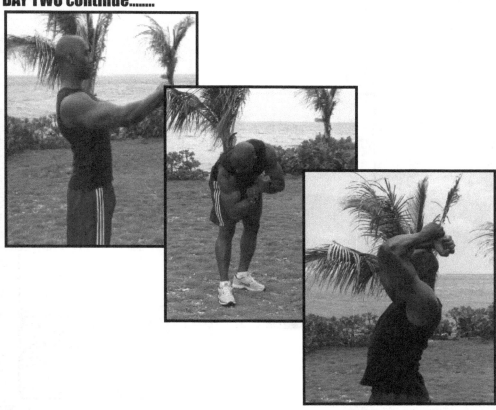

# THE ISOMETRIC 10,10,10 PROGRAM

## 16 THE ISOMETRIC 10,10,10 PROGRAM

### HOW TO PERFORM THIS ROUTINE:
### THE ISOMETRIC FAT LOSS PROGRAM

Perform this **ISOMETRIC WORKOUT**—by placing the muscle at the mid-point contracted position. Hold that contracted position for 10,10,10 seconds each before moving onto another contraction. Perform all exercises one after the other until all exercises are completed without rest. Perform 3 rounds of these between each round rest for 10 seconds before starting the round again.
**Alternate day one and day two for 6 days per week.**
**DAY TWO continued..........**

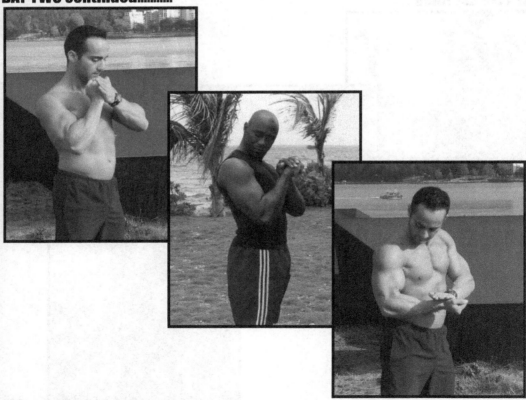

# THE ISOMETRIC 10,10,10 PROGRAM

## 16 THE ISOMETRIC 10,10,10 PROGRAM

### HOW TO PERFORM THIS ROUTINE:
### THE ISOMETRIC FAT LOSS PROGRAM

Perform this **ISOMETRIC WORKOUT**—by placing the muscle at the mid-point contracted position. Hold that contracted position for 10,10,10 seconds each before moving onto another contraction. Perform all exercises one after the other until all exercises are completed without rest. Perform 3 rounds of these between each round rest for 10 seconds before starting the round again.

**Alternate day one and day two for 6 days per week.**
**DAY TWO continued...........**

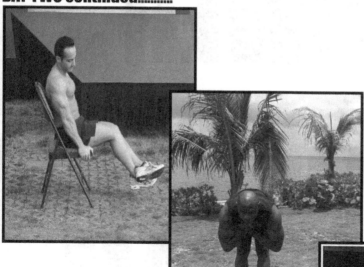

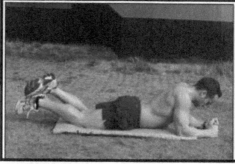

# Chapter 17

# THE ISOMETRIC POWER CONTRACTION PROGRAM

# THE ISOMETRIC POWER CONTRACTION PROGRAM

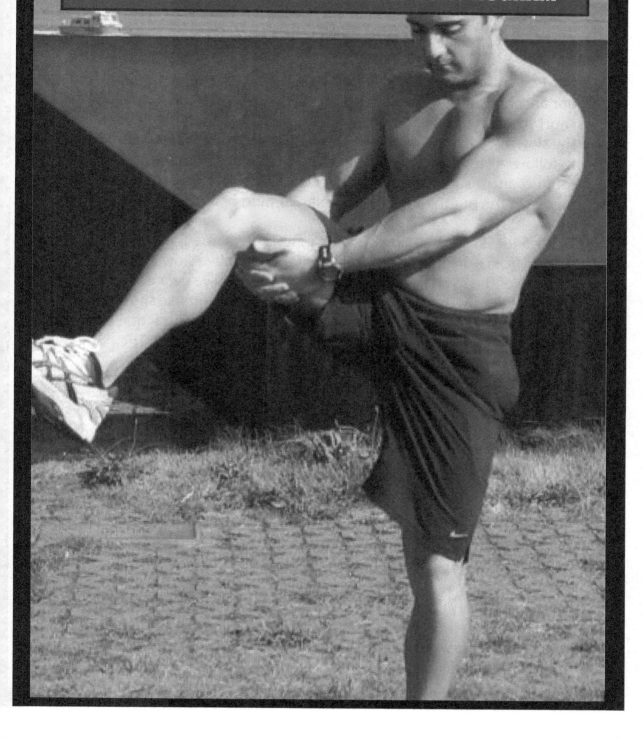

# THE ISOMETRIC POWER CONTRACTION PROGRAM

## 17 THE ISOMETRIC POWER CONTRACTION PROGRAM

The Power Isometric Contraction Method is an awesome size and defination enhancer because the trainee can perform loads of mini-contractions in a short space of time—and the first few mini-reps do a great job of fatiguing the slow-twitch fibers for more growth-fiber activation on the following reps to follow. All it takes is two to three rounds, that's a serious muscle-building routine; and it should take you less than 20 minutes. This routine muscle blast increases the pump in the fibers while burning bodyfat.

The trainee is also cranking out a lot of reps in a short space of time, but the sets go from ridiculously easy feeling (for cumulative slow-twitch fatigue) to some of the most intense full blown pumps you've ever done this really stimulates (growth-fiber-activation). The key is the intense short mini-contraction reps that lasts between 1-2 seconds per contraction this adds cumulative fatigue, as well as volume of (20 plus mini-reps). The pump will be super crazy and off the charts.

**Here's how it is done:**

Let's use the classic Liederman contraction for an example, start off as shown in the picture (press) the hands together pause for 1-2 seconds, release the pressure for 1second and continue for 20 mini-contractions).

After the mini contractions, hold for a count of 20 seconds on top of that. As stated before, the first set will be easy—very easy to be honest.

However, the key is that you are creating cumulative fatigue in the targeted muscle, and the first few reps are fatiguing the slow-twitch fibers, due to the volume of blood, lactic acid buildup and hormonal release that takes place.

# THE ISOMETRIC POWER CONTRACTION PROGRAM

## 17 THE ISOMETRIC POWER CONTRACTION PROGRAM

By the second set you will be feeling it more than ever. Endurance slow-twitch fibers are starting to burnout, then the fast-twitch endurance fibers begin firing rapidly, and by the 20th rep you will have trouble completing those last few reps due to the intense muscle burn. This really push those endurance fast-twitch fibers for optimum fat-burning and enhanced growth. Isometric pulses works because it targets the motor units hard, coaxing them to rapidly fire mini reps that increases blood volume, lactic acid buildup and hormonal fat-burning properties.

This hits multiple fiber types, and increases tension over-load due to the mini-pulses which will fatigue the endurance fast and slow-twitch fibers, creating intense muscle fiber activation on the muscles involved. While waking up the dormant fibers to fire rapidly. This Isometric Power Program will coax more muscle stimulation to more muscle fibers than "traditional" high tension isometric low second contractions. This Program of isometric contraction will lead to a greater degree of lean muscular development.

In other words, moderate tension coupled with extended load time will coax more muscle-building-effects. This activates the target muscle significantly greater and enhances endurance-oriented-fast-twitch muscle fibers to promote muscular growth and strength rapidly.

# THE ISOMETRIC POWER CONTRACTION PROGRAM

## 17 THE ISOMETRIC POWER CONTRACTION PROGRAM

The primary mechanisms for muscle growth and how they correlate to The Isometric Power Contraction Program are:

1)Continuous tension which increases metabolic stress with contraction type exercises, this blocks blood flow, due to the nature of the exercise and the element of tension being on the muscle's trigger spot.

2)Some exercises increase the muscle's length but resistance is maintained throughout the muscle. This increases various hormonal production which coax the fat-burning effects.

Using the Isometric Power Program stimulates the primary mechanics for increasing muscle and fat burning stimulation. By increasing time under load this pre-fatigue the slow-twitch fibers, which enhances an extraordinary amount of endurance fast twitch fibers to fire rapidly.  The Isometric Power Program is a great multi-fat-burning system. That not only burn bodyfat, but increases lean musculature threefold.

The routine hammers away at your muscles within minutes by alternating various muscle groups which receive an accelerated recovery boast because the other muscles are resting or being stretched. For instance when you do a across-the body row, this pre-stretch the chest muscles, but cause the upper back and rear delts contract.

Plus, when an isometric curl is performed, your tricep go into an elongated state every time the biceps contract and the same for the triceps. This actually helps the muscles recharge it's batteries for upcoming sets.

# THE ISOMETRIC POWER CONTRACTION PROGRAM

## 17 THE ISOMETRIC POWER CONTRACTION PROGRAM

The Isometric Power Contraction Program is an extra fiber activating enhancer. You will experience that longer tension times coax more growth fibers to fire on extended power contraction reps that follow.
The program builds successful muscle growth due to tension overload with this high rep load technique, you accomplish a lot of workload within a short time frame.

In other words, you will be training each bodypart more frequently through out the week for a more massively hard as nails ripped physique. This brings us to The Isometric Power Contraction Method.

# THE ISOMETRIC POWER CONTRACTION PROGRAM

## 17 THE ISOMETRIC POWER CONTRACTION PROGRAM

### HOW TO PERFORM THIS ROUTINE:
### THE ISOMETRIC POWER CONTRACTION PROGRAM

Perform the **ISOMETRIC POWER CONTRACTION WORKOUT**—at the contracted position pictured pause for 1-2 seconds, release the pressure 1 inch and continue for 20 more mini-contractions (**NON-STOP**). After the mini contractions, hold for a count of 20 seconds. Perform all exercises without rest for 2 rounds.

**Alternate day one and day two for 6 days per week for 2 weeks**
**DAY ONE**

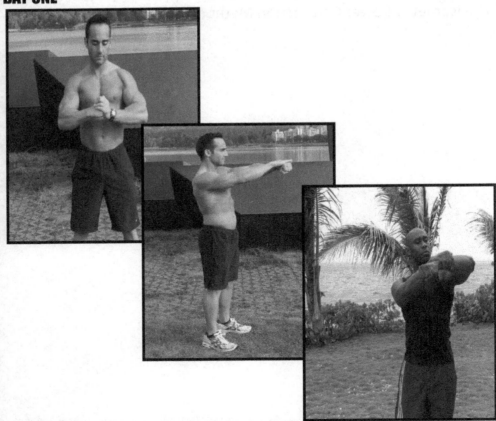

# THE ISOMETRIC POWER CONTRACTION PROGRAM

## 17 THE ISOMETRIC POWER CONTRACTION PROGRAM

**HOW TO PERFORM THIS ROUTINE:**
**THE ISOMETRIC POWER CONTRACTION PROGRAM**

Perform the **ISOMETRIC POWER CONTRACTION WORKOUT**—at the contracted position pictured pause for 1-2 seconds, release the pressure 1 inch and continue for 20 more mini-contractions (**NON-STOP**). After the mini contractions, hold for a count of 20 seconds. Perform all exercises without rest for 2 rounds.

**Alternate day one and day two for 6 days per week for 2 weeks**
**DAY ONE continued..........**

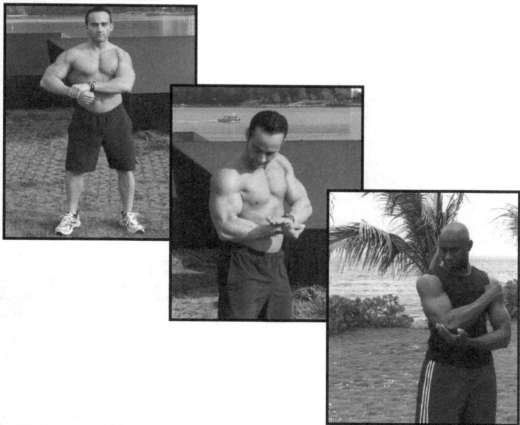

# THE ISOMETRIC POWER CONTRACTION PROGRAM

## 17  THE ISOMETRIC POWER CONTRACTION PROGRAM

### HOW TO PERFORM THIS ROUTINE:
### THE ISOMETRIC POWER CONTRACTION PROGRAM

Perform the **ISOMETRIC POWER CONTRACTION WORKOUT**—at the contracted position pictured pause for 1-2 seconds, release the pressure 1 inch and continue for 20 more mini-contractions (**NON-STOP**). After the mini contractions, hold for a count of 20 seconds. Perform all exercises without rest for 2 rounds.

**Alternate day one and day two for 6 days per week for 2 weeks**
**DAY ONE continued..........**

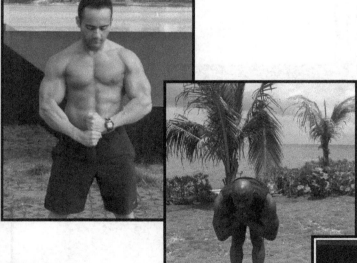

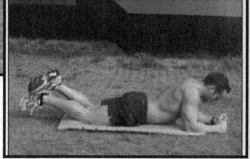

# THE ISOMETRIC POWER CONTRACTION PROGRAM

## 17 THE ISOMETRIC POWER CONTRACTION PROGRAM

### HOW TO PERFORM THIS ROUTINE:
### THE ISOMETRIC POWER CONTRACTION PROGRAM

Perform the **ISOMETRIC POWER CONTRACTION WORKOUT**—at the contracted position pictured pause for 1-2 seconds, release the pressure 1 inch and continue for 20 more mini-contractions (**NON-STOP**). After the mini contractions, hold for a count of 20 seconds.  Perform all exercises without rest for 2 rounds.

**Alternate day one and day two for 6 days per week for 2 weeks**
**DAY TWO**

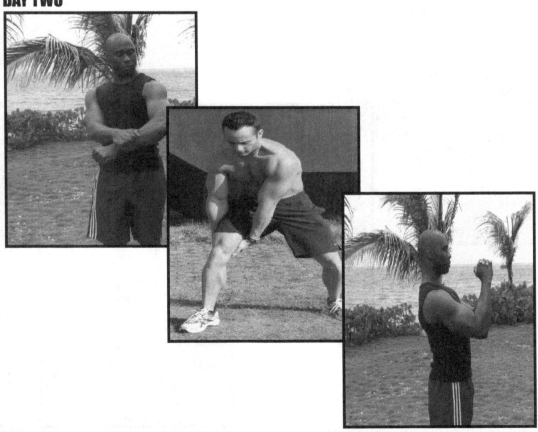

# THE ISOMETRIC POWER PULSE PROGRAM

## 17 THE ISOMETRIC POWER CONTRACTION PROGRAM

### HOW TO PERFORM THIS ROUTINE:
### THE ISOMETRIC POWER CONTRACTION PROGRAM

Perform the **ISOMETRIC POWER CONTRACTION WORKOUT**—at the contracted position pictured pause for 1-2 seconds, release the pressure 1 inch and continue for 20 more mini-contractions (**NON-STOP**). After the mini contractions, hold for a count of 20 seconds on top of that. Perform all exercises without rest for 2 rounds.
**Alternate day one and day two for 6 days per week for 2 weeks
DAY TWO continued...........**

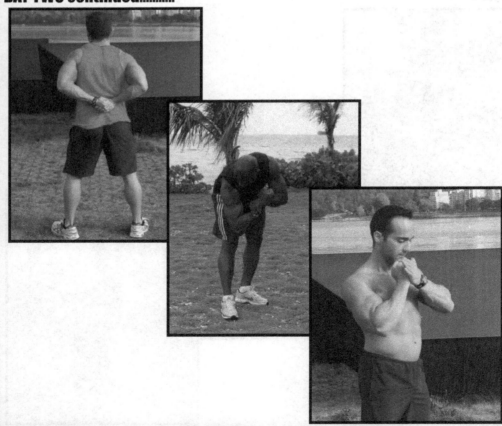

# THE ISOMETRIC POWER PULSE PROGRAM

# 17 THE ISOMETRIC POWER CONTRACTION PROGRAM

## HOW TO PERFORM THIS ROUTINE:
## THE ISOMETRIC POWER CONTRACTION PROGRAM

Perform the **ISOMETRIC POWER CONTRACTION WORKOUT**—at the contracted position pictured pause for 1-2 seconds, release the pressure 1 inch and continue for 20 more mini-contractions (**NON-STOP**). After the mini contractions, hold for a count of 20 seconds. Perform all exercises without rest for 2 rounds.

**Alternate day one and day two for 6 days per week for 2 weeks**
**DAY TWO continued...........**

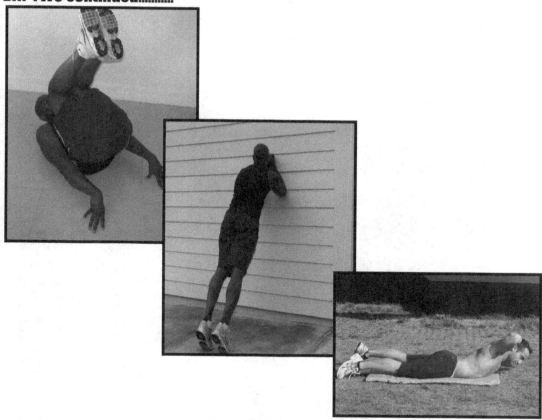

**W**e are looking forward to hearing from you on your progress. Please drop us an email isometricskiwi@gmail.com and skippymarl@icloud.com

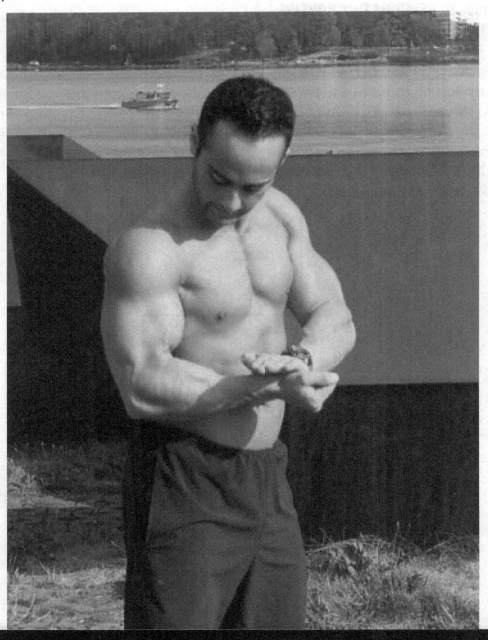

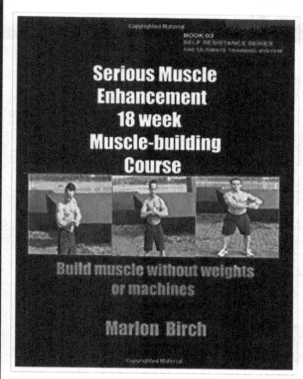

# Pack on pounds of muscle fast!

**BUILD MUSCLES WITHOUT WEIGHTS** Self Resistance when done correctly, will sculpt, reshape and add strength to a person's physique beyond imagination without the use of weights or machines. The Serious Muscle Enhancement Program is the official Self-Resistance muscle-sculpting manual with full-range body-part workouts for every major muscle, with plenty of training tips and tricks to get you building muscles fast.

Learn how to get maximum muscle fiber recruitment and full-muscle development without weights for every body part at every workout. There's a full look at my 18-pound-of-muscle-in-12-weeks original program, and the changes I made to improve the stress methods and results.

You get an innovative muscle-sculpting and strength workout plan without ever having to go to a gym or lift weights. This manual is an absolute must for your muscle-building library, and it's the cornerstone from which most of my programs were created that will take your physique into the fourth dimension!

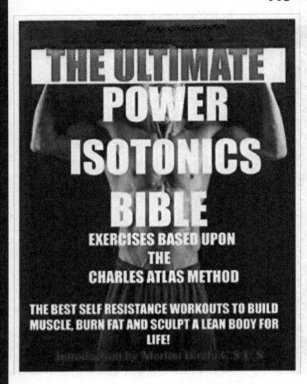

**P**owerful routines to get in shape!

**THE ULTIMATE POWER ISOTONICS BIBLE** THE BEST SELF RESISTANCE WORK-OUTS TO BUILD MUSCLE,BURN FAT AND SCULPT A LEAN BODY FOR LIFE!

Do it anywhere, any time, it is the perfect exercise plan all without weights and machines. Build the body of your dreams today. The unique muscle-building exercises in this book will get you growing like crazy because they push your muscles with muscle-building-enhancing exercises and routines with–60 to 90 seconds of tension, which muscles need to increase strength and size.

In this easy-to-read book, you will see illustrations that explain each pro gram—and you will finally see why almost everyone is doing self resistance wrong and why their growth is so painfully slow—Marlon Birch knows the "secrets" on getting amazing muscle size and strength in record time.

He is the ONLY self resistance trainer to take the original Charles Atlas type exercises, enhance them in Hy-brid fashion and became the first ever Professional Bodybuilder using only these exercises to accomplish that goal. Learn from the world's respected fitness trainer and 3-time natural pro body builder be your personal trainer today.

# COMING SOON
# 20TH JULY 2019
# TRANSFORMATION CONTEST!

Make a purchase of any of these books save your recite to get a chance to win $$$$$. Contact skippymarl@icloud.com email title (**CONTEST**) Announcements on the way stay tuned.

Printed in May 2022
by Rotomail Italia S.p.A., Vignate (MI) - Italy